THE
HERB GROWER'S
GRIMOIRE

Traditional Recipes,
Herbal Wisdom, & Ancient Lore

'It is impossible to describe to one who does not feel by instinct "the lure of green things growing" the curious stimulation, the sense of intoxication, of delight, brought about by working among such green-growing, sweet scented things.'

– **Alice Morse Earle,** *Old Time Gardens,* **1901**

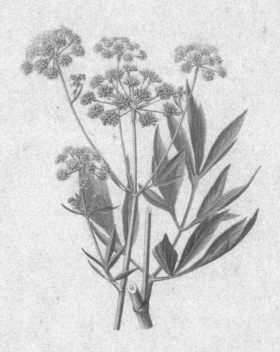

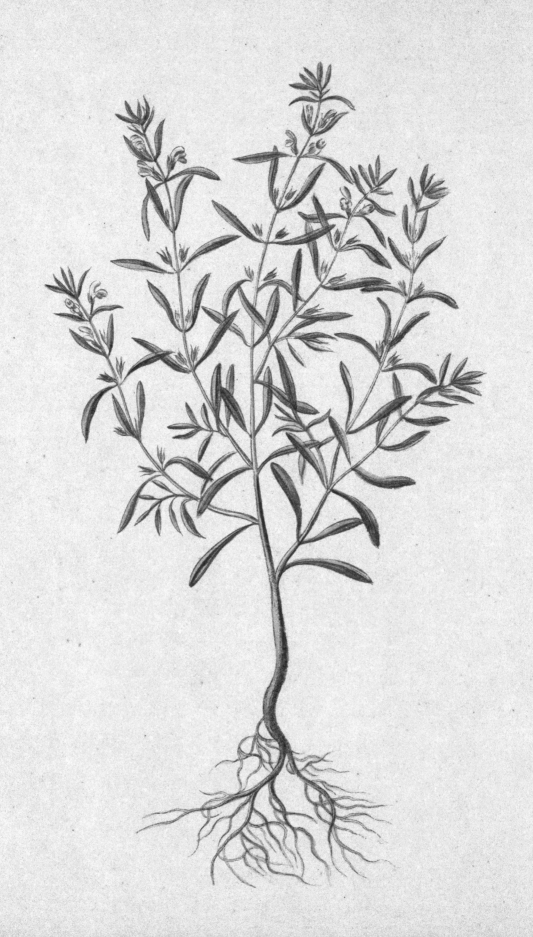

CONTENTS

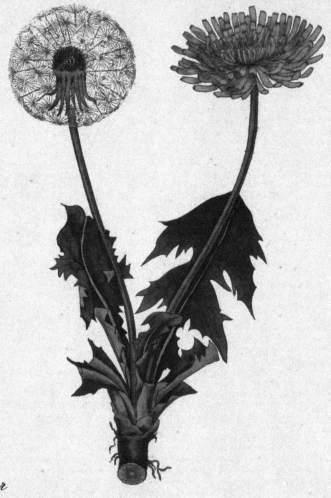

Disclaimer

The information in this volume has been collected from a breadth of sources on the subject of herbalism. Our information is sourced from an array of ancient writings by Roman philosophers, nineteenth-century farming almanacks, and beautifully illustrated herbals penned across centuries — capturing a unique picture of the herbal field. We have chosen to include much of the the original language as it was published, with the older sources hailing vocabulary from centuries past. You will find a glossary of terms at the back of the volume.

While we have carefully produced a book that includes practical uses for everyday herbs, the reader must be aware of the historical context in which the original sources were written. We have ensured that most recipes, remedies, spells, and charms featured in this book are not harmful, however, such antiquated information must be regarded within the temporal setting of their first publication, and any medicinal remedies or suggestions should only be acted upon with the consultation of a medical professional, especially those pregnant or breast feeding. We have incorporated some of the more obscure extracts as examples of the arcane lore that laid the foundations of modern herbalist practice, although they are not included as practical remedies or information for actual use.

INTRODUCTION

Planting, growing, and gathering herbs has been a common practice for centuries, with gardens artfully tailored to produce a myriad of herbs for personal use. Many of our common herbs were once abundantly harvested for their properties, often utilised for medicinal, nutritional, and even magical virtues. While such a holistic method of harnessing the power of herbs may have been forgotten in the modern age, the enchanting natural lore at the heart of herbalist practice is preserved in books left unread and in the stories passed from generation to generation.

The Herb Grower's Grimoire is a carefully curated volume of lost herbal knowledge, folklore, and ancient wisdom for thirty of the most common garden herbs. Split into two sections, this volume's first half delves into the history of herbs, covering subjects such as herbs in cooking, medicine, magic, and astrology, as well as how to plant, grow, harvest, and store herbs for such purposes. In the second half, you will find a list of common herbs and plants. Under each, key botanical information is listed along with practical advice on growing and gathering. Details of culinary properties and medicinal and magical virtues have been collated, as well as ingots of folklore, herbal charms, and legends specific to each herb. By blending the practical with the whimsical, and often romantic, this book offers a unique look at the landscape of ancient herbalist practice. Its pages bring to light the forgotten stories each herb holds while providing hands-on advice for application of older herbal knowledge in a contemporary setting.

Although this volume is not solely dedicated to magical practice, the titular term 'grimoire' is an intrinsic expression of the collected wisdom herein. A grimoire is defined as a spell book or textbook of magic, taken from the old French *grammaire*. The term once referred to all books written in Latin, however, by the eighteenth century it had evolved to define texts on magic and later became a figure of speech to describe something hard to understand, often with ties to the occult. While the lore of herbs is intrinsically linked to mystical and esoteric practices, there also lies a magic in the timeless methods of cultivating, gathering, and harvesting herbs. The unmistakable lure of the garden and the joyful act of growing from seed or cutting can be as enchanting as the charms, remedies, and beliefs that infuse herbalism itself.

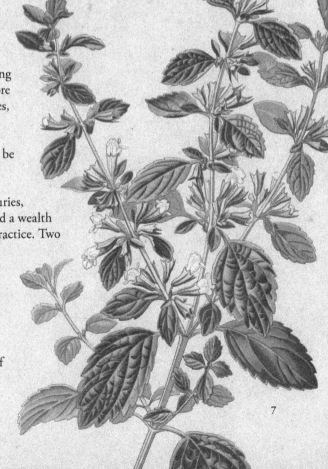

If we turn to the fifteenth, sixteenth, and seventeenth centuries, often regarded as the great ages of herbal remedies, we can find a wealth of knowledge that helped form modern ideas around herbal practice. Two cornerstone herbals in the English language, John Gerard's *The Herball; or, Generall Historie of Plantes* (1597) and Nicholas Culpeper's *The English Physician Enlarged* (1653), forged the landscape for traditional herbal healing among the masses. They delivered insightful information on the uses of herbs for healing in an artful blend of conventional medicine, astrology, magic, and folklore. For instance, Culpeper's medicinal suggestion for applying basil to the stings or bites of venomous creatures to draw out the poison is followed by a

INTRODUCTION

story about a man who, upon smelling the herb, had a scorpion grow on his brain. Culpeper ties this association with poisonous creatures to basil's attribution to the planet Mars, which resides in the house of Scorpio in astrological lore. Ancient herbalists assigned herbs to specific planetary rulers based on their unique attributes and growing season, and as seen in Culpeper's work, the herbs gained the properties and characteristics associated with those planets, which were also considered when administering herbs for health.

Astrological factors influenced the medicinal remedies further through the linkage of the twelve signs of the zodiac to specific body parts. This practice dates back to as early as the 1300s, and the use of a standard image known as the 'Man of Signs' illustrated these associations. Commonly found on the pages of almanacks and herbals alike, the image depicts the body of a man, displaying the twelve astrological signs and their correlating body parts. This underlying current of celestial influence weaves its way throughout herbalism, with many of the core understandings being based on folkloric beliefs of higher powers. Established centuries before modern medicine, these ideologies forged the foundation of herbal medicine, although the remedies often, and unsurprisingly, fell short of their promise.

Ancient physicians such as Dioscorides and Galen outlined the medicinal uses of herbs in the Doctrine of Signatures, established around 200 AD. This theory states the specific healing purposes of each plant and proposes that the shape of a herb is directly linked to a corresponding body part that shares a similar form. For example, the heart-shaped mint leaves were believed to treat cardiovascular issues, while lung-shaped plants like sage and comfrey were applied for pulmonary complaints. Much of the knowledge compiled in the old herbals was gathered from ancient writings like those of Pliny the Elder (Roman author and naturalist philosopher), Dioscorides, and Galen. They were heavily referenced throughout the centuries, forming the basis of modern herbal knowledge. As Gerard writes in his 1653 work, 'The leaves and flowers of Borrage put into wine make men and women glad and merry, driving away all sadness, dullness, and melancholy, as Dioscorides and Pliny affirm.'

The stories passed down through the generations inform much of the narrative now surrounding herbs and their uses. Since the fifteenth-century herbals, practical remedies have been woven with myths and legends from ancient Greece, superstitions and charms from days gone by, as well as herb-specific planting rituals and growing advice from across the globe. This sense of the supernatural infusing the herbalist practice has been present since immemorial. From being worn as amulets, offering protection and good fortune to the wearer, to being used as key ingredients in spells and rituals, herbs have been used in magical and spiritual practices. While they can vary from culture to culture, there remains a common belief that certain herbs carry unique energies and powers. Writing of rue in *A Modern Herbal* (1913), Maude Grieve speaks of how it was regarded by the ancient Greeks as an 'anti-magical herb', as it failed to treat nervous indigestion felt before meeting strangers, which they attributed to witchcraft. Many of the old notions of herbal magic may now seem overtly romantic, such as pinning bay leaves to the four corners of a pillow in the hope of dreaming of a future beloved, there are elements of

INTRODUCTION

mystical beliefs that remain. Garlic was once believed to be an effective repellent of dark magic. It was commonly hung up in households as a protective amulet, similarly to garlic bulbs being worn to ward off vampires in modern literature.

In this volume, we have included many of the remedies and charms featuring herbs as vital ingredients, yet we have omitted some of the more obscure beliefs, cures, and spells from past centuries as they are now unbefitting for the modern age. The following medicinal remedy from Pliny's *Natural History* (c. 77 AD) prescribes nettle seeds 'taken in the broth of a boiled tortoise' as an antidote for salamander and serpent bites, henbane poison, and scorpion stings. Even more arcane, and not included in this volume for obvious reasons, is the Welsh belief that a human skull, grated like one would the root of ginger and mixed with a liquid, was believed to be a sufficient remedy against fits. When placed in a contemporary context, such treatments highlight the folkloric heart of the herbalist practice, and while many of them may seem ridiculous to today's reader, these remedies and spells held real gravitas in an age before modern medicine and science.

Just as elements of ancient herbal knowledge endure, so do some of the primordial methods of sowing, cultivating, and harvesting herbs. Before the days of horticultural science, when herbology was at its most popular, many gardeners established their techniques around the natural cycle of the Earth and her seasons, turning again to planetary forces for guidance. One unique gardening style suggested that growing herbs according to the moon's lunar cycle would help increase the quality and growth of the garden's bounty. As James George Frazer writes in *The Golden Bough* (1911), 'In various parts of Europe it is believed that plants (…) cut while the moon is on the increase, will grow again fast, but that if cut while it is on the decrease they will grow slowly or waste away.' While growing by the moon may seem to some a whimsical method, modern science has proven the influence of the moon's cycle on the push and pull of water on Earth, with many gardeners harnessing its powers in their planting calendar. Much like the tides, the moon's energy affects the movement of water beneath the soil's surface, bringing but also taking away water from the roots of plants, with the ability to both aid and harbour growing success.

The influence of higher powers was believed to affect not only the planting of herbs but also the harvesting, drying, and administering processes. Since the days of Odin, picking ceremonies have permeated the methods of herbalist practice, being closely intertwined with broader religions and belief systems. Ancient traditions of gathering herbs for noble purposes involved the worship of the Earth and of gods and goddesses of nature. Later, prayers and picking ceremonies were incorporated into these practices, often with the intention of renouncing the devil and dark forces. There was an Irish belief that some herbs became malefic if broken by hand, becoming prime ingredients for those practising dark magic. It was also believed that others held sacred healing properties if they were gathered on May Day and picked in the name of the Holy Trinity.

Many of the rituals and ceremonies for gathering herbs focus on the magical effects of higher powers on the plants' virtues. At the same time, the physical act of harvesting in season is dictated by the growing cycle of each, and with the cultivation of herbs being a fundamental part of the holistic cycle and application of herbalism, it is essential to include the long-established traditions and advice on creating and nurturing a thriving herb garden. We must remember that one of the core fundamentals of the herb garden was to provide sustenance for the household above all else, with herbs grown abundantly in kitchen gardens. They have been used in cooking and recipes across the globe for centuries, threading their way through the core of the world's cuisines and cultures. Herbs are commonly applied to season and elevate dishes, whether picked fresh or dried, and they often provide added nutritional benefits.

Mapping the intrinsic ties herbs have with the history of human culture through their botanical, medicinal, astrological, and folkloric virtues, herbalists have harnessed the appeal of the natural world and all the wonders it beholds. *The Herb Grower's Grimoire* is a rich resource for even the most amateur gardener, detailing aspects of traditional gardening to establish and nurture an abundant and beneficial plot. In this book, each herb is accompanied by practical growing advice for the modern garden, along with its planting and harvesting months, companion plants, and recipes for use in the kitchen.

The curious history of herbs will spark intrigue for centuries to come, and the mindful cycle of planting, growing, eating, and utilising herbs for their properties will continue. We hope this unique volume of forgotten herbal wisdom, recipes, and folklore will act as another stepping stone in preserving and passing on this indispensable knowledge from one generation to the next. With any luck, the stories of these herbs will live on long after we are gone.

INTRODUCTION

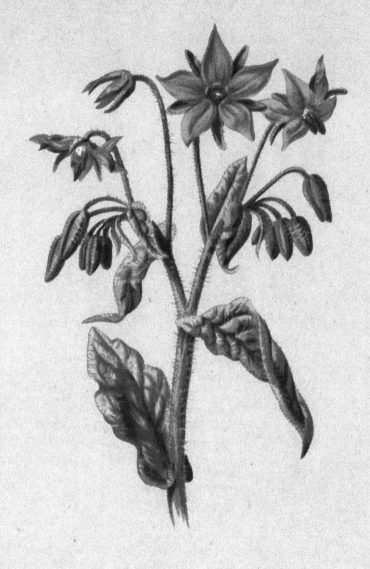

A chaplet then of Herbs I'll make
Than which though yours be braver,
Yet this of mine I'll undertake
Shall not be short in savour.
With Basil then I will begin,
Whose scent is wondrous pleasing:
This Eglantine I'll next put in
The sense with sweetness seizing.
Then in my Lavender I lay
Muscado put among it,
With here and there a leaf of Bay,
Which still shall run along it.
Germander, Marjoram and Thyme,
Which uséd are for strewing;
With Hyssop as an herb most prime
Here in my wreath bestowing.
Then Balm and Mint help to make up
My chaplet, and for trial
Costmary that so likes the Cup,
And next it Pennyroyal.
Then Burnet shall bear up with this,
Whose leaf I greatly fancy;
Some Camomile doth not amiss
With Savory and some Tansy.
Then here and there I'll put a sprig
Of Rosemary into it,
Thus not too Little nor too Big,
'Tis done if I can do it.

– Michael Drayton, *The Muses Elizium,* **1630**

Again, what other plants have such a remarkable literature as herbs? The
old herbals and gardening books are a source of profound interest not only
to gardeners and botanists but also to artists, folklorists, ethnologists, and
philologists. To some of us no small part of the pleasure of wandering in the pages
of these books is due to the charm of the writers' personalities.

– Eleanour Sinclair Rohde, *Herbs and Herb Gardening,* **1936**

HISTORY OF HERBS IN MEDICINE & MAGIC

The humbler art of Medicine chose
The knowledge of each plant that grows.

– Virgil, Aeneid: XII, c. 19 BC

The Lord has created medicines out of the earth; and he that is wise will not abhor them.

– Ecclesiasticus 38:4 King James Bible

Healing by herbs has always been popular both with the classic nations of old, and with the British islanders of more recent times. Two hundred and sixty years before the date of Hippocrates (460 B.C.) the prophet Isaiah bade King Hezekiah, when sick unto death, "take a lump of Figs, and lay it on the boil; and straightway the King recovered."

Lapis, the favourite pupil of Apollo, was offered endowments of skill in augury, music, or archery. But he preferred to acquire a knowledge of herbs for service of cure in sickness; and, armed with this knowledge, he saved the life of Aeneas when grievously wounded by an arrow. He averted the hero's death by applying the plant "Dittany," smooth of leaf, and purple of blossom, as plucked on the mountain Ida.

It is told in Malvern Chase that Mary of Eldersfield (1454), "whom some called a witch," famous for her knowledge of herbs and medicaments, "descending the hill from her hut, with a small phial of oil, and a bunch of the 'Danewort,' speedily enabled Lord Edward of March, who had just then heavily sprained his knee, to avoid danger by mounting 'Roan Roland' freed from pain, as it were by magic, through the plant-rubbing which Mary administered."

In Shakespeare's time there was a London street, named Bucklersbury (near the present Mansion House), noted for its number of druggists who sold Simples and sweet-smelling herbs. We read, in *The Merry Wives of Windsor*, that Sir John Falstaff flouted the effeminate fops of his day as "Lisping hawthorn buds that smell like Bucklersbury in simple time."

Various British herbalists have produced works, more or less learned and voluminous, about our native medicinal plants

– William Thomas Fernie, Herbal Simples: Approved for Modern Uses of Cure, 1897

O who can tell The hidden power of herbes and might of Magicke spell?

– Edmund Spenser, The Fairie Queene, 1590

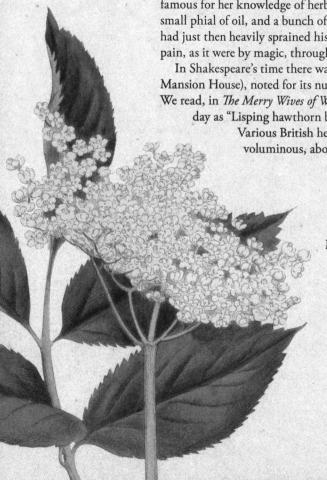

HISTORY OF HERBS IN
MEDICINE & MAGIC

In a herb garden we look as it were through magic casements into a past strangely different from this material and mechanized age. Some of the humblest herbs carry us back in thought to the dim past ages pictured in the oldest parts of Widsith and Beowulf, and to centuries when healing herbs were gathered with ceremonies associated with forms of religion so ancient that compared to them the worship of Woden is modern. Urban and suburban life have deprived the masses of our people not only of their birthright of forests, meadows, and fields, but the vast majority have never had even a glimpse of Nature in her untamed strength and grandeur. But herbs recall the centuries when Nature reigned supreme in these islands and the few scattered hamlets were on the verge of vast uninhabited stretches of country. We are reminded of our ancestors' beliefs in supernatural beings who infested the trackless wastes and impenetrable forests and of their belief in herbs to quell these powers of evil. For to these supernatural beings, always at enmity with mankind, were ascribed many of the ills to which flesh is heir. Some herbs were held so sacred they could be gathered only when the stars were auspicious and with prayers strangely intermingled with heathen incantations. Not a few of these incantations, such as "Nine were Nonnes sisters", preserved in the eleventh century Saxon Lacnunga, are curiously suggestive of children's counting-out games.

– **Eleanour Sinclair Rohde**, *Herbs and Herb Gardening*, 1936

The Art of Simpling

Herb gardens were no vanity and no luxury in our grandmothers' day; they were a necessity. To them every good housewife turned for nearly all that gave variety to her cooking, and to fill her domestic pharmacopœia. The physician placed his chief reliance for supplies on herb gardens and the simples of the fields. An old author says, "Many an old wife or country woman doth often more good with a few known and common garden herbs, than our bombast physicians, with all their prodigious, sumptuous, far-fetched, rare, conjectural medicines." Doctor and goodwife both had a rival in the parson. The picture of the country parson and his wife given by old George Herbert was equally true of the New England minister and his wife:—

"In the knowledge of simples one thing would be carefully observed, which is to know what herbs may be used instead of drugs of the same nature, and to make the garden the shop; for home-bred medicines are both more easy for the parson's purse, and more familiar for all men's bodies. So when the apothecary useth either for loosing Rhubarb, or for binding Bolearmana,

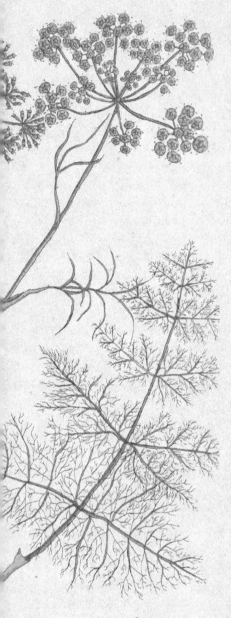

the parson useth damask or white Rose for the one, and Plantain, Shepherd's Purse, and Knot-grass for the other; and that with better success. As for spices, he doth not only prefer home-bred things before them, but condemns them for vanities, and so shuts them out of his family, esteeming that there is no spice comparable for herbs to Rosemary, Thyme, savory Mints, and for seeds to Fennel and Caraway. Accordingly, for salves, (...) his wife seeks not the city, but prefers her gardens and fields before all outlandish gums."

Simples were medicinal plants, so called because each of these vegetable growths was held to possess an individual virtue, to be an element, a simple substance constituting a single remedy. The noun was generally used in the plural.

You must not think that sowing, gathering, drying, and saving these herbs and simples in any convenient or unstudied way was all that was necessary. Not at all; many and manifold were the rules just when to plant them, when to pick them, how to pick them, how to dry them, and even how to keep them. Gervayse Markham was very wise in herb lore, in the suited seasons of the moon, and hour of the day or night, for herb culling.

(...)

Thomas Tusser wrote:—

"Good huswives provide, ere an sickness do come, Of sundrie good things in house to have some, Good aqua composita, vinegar tart, Rose water and treacle to comfort the heart, Good herbes in the garden for agues that burn, That over strong heat to good temper turn."

(...)

From herbs and simples were made, for internal use, liquid medicines such as wines and waters, syrups, juleps; and solids, such as conserves, confections, treacles, eclegms, tinctures. There were for external use, amulets, oils, ointments, liniments, plasters, cataplasms, salves, poultices; also sacculi, little bags of flowers, seeds, herbs, etc., and pomanders and posies.

– Alice Morse Earle, *Old Time Gardens*, 1901

Ancient people used to divine future events, victory in wars, safety in a dangerous voyage, triumph of a projected undertaking, success in love, recovery from sickness, or the approach of death; all through the skilful use of herbs, the knowledge of which had come down to them through the earliest traditions of the human race.

– Jane Wilde, *Ancient Legends, Mystic Charms and Superstitions of Ireland*, 1919

HISTORY OF HERBS IN MEDICINE & MAGIC

The art of *Simpling* is as old with us as our British hills. It aims at curing common ailments with simple remedies culled from the soil, or at home from resources near at hand.

Since the days of the anglo-saxons such remedies have been chiefly herbal; insomuch that the word "drug" came originally from their verb *drigan*, to dry, as applied to medicinal plants. These primitive Simplers were guided in their choice of herbs partly by watching animals who sought them out for self-cure, and partly by discovering for themselves the sensible properties of the plants as revealed by their odour and taste ; also by their supposed resemblance to those diseases which nature meant them to heal.

– William Thomas Fernie, *Herbal Simples: Approved for Modern Uses of Cure*, 1897

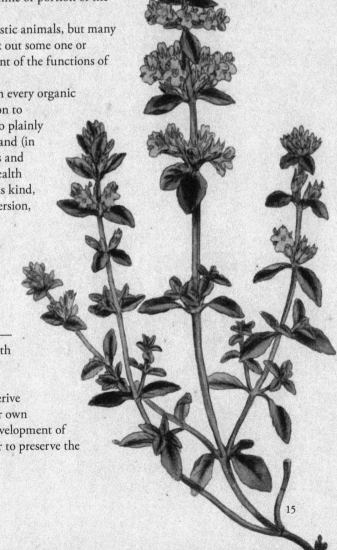

From the many facts existing, we must believe that there is not a single disease in man that may not have its remedy or cure, in some herb or other, if we but knew which plant, and where to find it, in this, or that, or any clime or portion of the world — agreeably to the providence of Nature.

(...) who has not often seen not only our familiar domestic animals, but many of the untamed creatures of the forests, fields, and air, seek out some one or peculiar herb, when laboring under sickness or derangement of the functions of its organism?

Truly, Nature has wisely implanted a definite instinct in every organic creature, in order to serve for its health, or for its restoration to health from disease. In man, however, such in fact is not so plainly marked, but to him has been given reason and judgment, and (in some feign of the race) a disposition to investigate the laws and mysteries of creation, in order to secure his own highest health and perfection, and to find the means for the healing of his kind, when they have become diseased through ignorance, perversion, and violation of the immutable ordinances of Creation.

As the proverb says, "There are sermons in stones, and books in running brooks;" so do we behold volumes of wisdom in all the herbal kingdom— in every emerald and variegated leaf, in every tinted blossom — in all there is a voiceless language, eternally singing significant psalms in Praise of "Him who doeth all things well."

Thus we find that adaptation is the law of the universe — and nowhere is it more vividly portrayed than in the growth and development of the Herbal world.

It will thus be seen that it is only by carefully studying the physiology or functions, or nature of plants, we can derive instruction for the proper regulation or government of our own organisms. The causes which influence the growth and development of plants, are conditions necessary to be understood, in order to preserve the health or integrity of our systems.

(...)

HISTORY OF HERBS IN
MEDICINE & MAGIC

Plants by their appearance often invite the invalid to cull them for his restoration, and assume such shapes as to suggest their curative properties. For instance, herbs that simulate the shape of the Lungs, as Lungwort, Sage, Hounds-tongue, and Comfrey, are all good for pulmonary complaints.

Plants which bear in leaves and roots a heart-like form, as Citron Apple, Fuller's Thistle, Spikenard, Balm, Mint, White-beet, Parsley, and Motherwort, will yield medicinal properties congenial to that organ. Vegetable productions like in figure to the ears as the leaves of the Coltfoot or Wild Spikenard, rightly prepared as a conserve and eaten, improve the hearing and memory... A decoction of Maiden Hair and the moss of Quinces, which plants resemble the hairs of the head, is good for baldness. Plants resembling the human nose as the leaves of the Wild Water Mint, are beneficial in restoring the sense of smell. Plants having a semblance of the Womb, as Birthwort, Heart Wort, Ladies' Seal or Briony, conduce much to a safe accouchement. Shrubs and Herbs resembling the bladder and gall, as Nightshade and Alkekengi, will relieve the gravel and stone. Liver-shaped plants, as Liverwort, Trinity, Agaric, Fumitory, Figs, etc., all are efficacious in bilious diseases. Walnuts, Indian nuts, Leeks, and the root of Ragwort, because of their form, when duly prepared will further generation and prevent sterility. Herbs and seeds in shape like the teeth, as Toothwort, Pine-kernel, etc., preserve the dental organization. Plants of knobbed form, like knuckles or joints, as Galingale, and the knotty odoriferous rush. Calamus, are good for diseases of the spine and reins, foot, gout, knee swellings, and all joint pains whatsoever. Oily vegetable products, as the Filbert, Walnut, Almond, etc., tend to fatness of the body (...) Fleshy plants, such as Onions, Leeks, and Cole wort, make flesh for the eaters. Certain plants, as the sensitive plant, Nettles, the roots of Mallows, and the herb Neurus, when used as outward applications, fortify and brace the nerves. Milky herbs, as Lettuce and the fruit of the Almond and Fig trees, propagate milk. Plants of a serious nature, as Spurge and Scammony, purge the noxious humors between the flesh and the skin. Herbs whose acidity turns milk to curd, such as Gallium and the seeds of Spurge, will lead to procreation. Rue mixed with Cumin will relieve a sore breast, if a poultice of them be applied, when the milk is knotted therein; while plants that are hollow, as the stalks of Grain, Reeds, Leeks, and Garlic, are good to purge, open, and soothe the hollow parts of the body.

– Nicholas Culpeper, *Complete Herbal,* 1824

HISTORY OF HERBS IN
MEDICINE & MAGIC

Herbal Magic & Lore

The vegetable world (…) has attracted writers since the earliest times, and in the days when supernatural agencies were almost always brought forward to account for un-comprehended phenomena, it was not marvellous that misty lore should lead to the association of plants and magic. The book of nature is not always easy to read, and the older students drew from it very personal interpretations. Some herbs were magical because they were used in spells and sorceries; others, because they had power in themselves. For instance, Basil, the perfume of which was thought to cause sympathy between two people, and in Moldavia they say it can even stop a wandering youth upon his way and make him love the maiden from whose hand he accepts a sprig. The Crocus flower, too, belongs to the second class, and brings laughter and great joy, and so it is with others. Plants were also credited with strong friendships and "enmities" amongst themselves. "The ancients" held strong views about their "sympathies and antipathies," and this sympathy or antipathy was attributed to individual likes and dislikes. "Rue dislikes Basil," says Pliny, "but Rue and the Fig-tree are in a great league and amitie" together. Alexanders loveth to grow in the same place as Rosemary, but the Radish is "at enmetie" with Hyssop. Savory and Onions are the better for each other's neighbourhood, and Coriander, Dill, Mallows, Herb-Patience and Chervil "love for companie to be set or sowne together." Bacon refers to some of these, but he took a prosaic view and thought these predilections due to questions of soil!

Being credited with such strong feelings amongst themselves, it is easier to understand how they were supposed to sympathise with their "environment." Honesty, of course, grew best in a very honest man's garden. Where Rosemary flourishes, the mistress rules. Sage will fade with the fortunes of the house and revive again as they recover; and Bay-trees are famous, but melancholy prophets.

> *Captain.*—'Tis thought the king is dead; we will not stay,
> The Bay-trees in our country are all wither'd. – *Richard II*. ii. iv.

From this, it is not a great step to acknowledge that particular plants have power to produce certain dispositions in the mind of man. So, the possession of a Rampion was likely to make a child quarrelsome: while, on the contrary, eating the leaves of Periwinkle "will cause love between a man and his wife." Laurel greatly "composed the phansy," and did "facilitate true visions," and was also "efficacious to inspire a poetical fury" (Evelyn). Having admitted the power of herbs over mental and moral qualities, we easily arrive at the recognition of their power in regard to the supernatural. If, as Culpepper tells us, "a raging bull, be he ever so mad, tied to a Fig-tree, will become tame and gentle;" or if, as Pliny says, any one, "by anointing himself with Chicory and oile will become right amiable and win grace and favour of all men, so that he shal the more easily obtain whatsoever his heart stands unto," it is not much wonder that St John's Wort would drive away tempests and evil spirits, four-leaved Clover enable the wearer to see witches, and Garlic avert the Evil Eye. Thus many herbs are magical "in their own right," so to speak, apart from those that are connected with magic, from being favourites of the fairies, the witches, and, in a few cases, the Evil One!

– **Rosalind Northcote,** *The Book of Herbs,* **1903**

The Influence of the Planets

The planets were another determining factor in the choice of remedies. Each plant was dedicated to a planet and each planet presided over a special part of the body, therefore, when any part was affected, a herb belonging to the planet that governed that special part must, as a rule, be used. Thus, Mercury presided over the brain, so for a headache (...) one of Mercury's herbs must be chosen. Mercurial herbs were, as a rule, refreshing, aromatic and of "very subtle parts." The planets seem usually to have caused, as well as cured the diseases in their special province, and therefore their own herbs, brought about the cure "by sympathy". But sometimes, a planet would cause a disorder in the province ruled by another planet, to whom the first was in opposition, and in this case the cure must be made "by antipathy." Thus the lungs are Jupiter, to whom Mercury is opposed, therefore in any case of the lungs being affected, the physician must first discover whether Jupiter or Mercury were the agent and if the latter, the remedy must be "antipathetical"; it must be from one of Mercury's herbs. Sometimes where a planet caused a disease in the part it governed, an "antipathetical" cure, by means of an adversary's herbs, was advised; for instance Jupiter is opposed to Saturn, so Jupiter's herbs might be given for toothache or pains in the bones caused by Saturn, for the bones were under Saturn's dominion. An antipathetical remedy, however, Culpeper does not recommend for common use, for "sympathetical cures strengthen nature; antipathetical cures, in one degree or another, weaken it." Besides this, the position of the planet had to be considered, the "House" that it was in, and the aspect in which it was to the moon and other planets. (...)

Turning to the Herbs appropriated to the special planets, we find that those of mars were usually strong, bright and vigorous, and cured ills caused by violence, including the sting of "a martial creature, imagine a wasp, a hornet, a scorpion." Yellow flowers were largely dedicated to the Sun or Moon, radiant, bright-yellow ones to the Sun; these of paler, fainter hues to the Moon. Flowers dedicated to either were good for the eyes, for the eyes are ruled by the "Luminaries." Jupiter's herbs had generally, "*Leaves* smooth, even, slightly cut and pointed, the veins not prominent. *Flowers* graceful, pleasing brights, succulent." The herbs of Venus were those with many flowers, of bright or delicate colours and pleasant odours. Saturn, who is almost always looked upon as being unfavourable, had only plants, whose leaves were "hairy, dry, hard, parched, coarse," and whose flowers were "gloomy, dull, greenish, faded or dirty white, pale red, invariably hirsute, prickly and disagreeable."

– **Rosalind Northcote,** *The Book of Herbs,* **1903**

HISTORY OF HERBS IN
MEDICINE & MAGIC

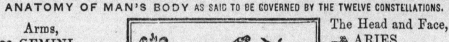

ANATOMY OF MAN'S BODY AS SAID TO BE GOVERNED BY THE TWELVE CONSTELLATIONS.

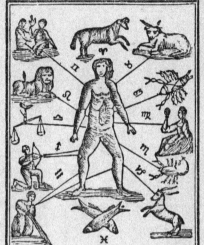

Arms,
GEMINI.

Heart,
LEO.

Reins,
LIBRA.

Thighs,
SAGITTARIUS

Legs,
AQUARIUS.

The Feet,
PISCES.

The Head and Face,
ARIES.

Neck,
TAURUS

Breast,
CANCER.

Bowels,
VIRGO.

Secrets,
SCORPIO.

Knees,
CAPRICORN.

– The Farmers Almanac For 1850, **1849**

The Man of Signs

The figure of a man, surrounded by the twelve Signs of the Zodiac, each referred to some part of his body by means of a connecting line or a pointing dagger, is still seen in some almanacs and was once regarded as indispensable. The Anatomy, as it was often called, was a graphic representation, intelligible alike to the educated and to those who could not read, of a vitally important principle in medicine and surgery. Each sign of the zodiac "governed" an organ or part of the body, and, in selecting a day to treat any ailment, or to let blood, it was necessary to know whether the moon was or was not in that sign.

(…)

It was a graphical summing up of the whole doctrine of astrological medicine. And medicine, for many centuries, had been permeated with astrology, both in theory and practice. Chaucer's physician in the Canterbury Tales always selected a fortunate ascendent in treating his patients, - that is, he observed the condition of the heavens, constructed a horoscope, and acted accordingly. Otherwise his ministrations might do more harm than good. Paracelsus declared, we are told, that no physician ought to write a prescription without consulting the stars. The science of one age becomes the superstition of the next, but what the Anatomy typified remained the doctrine of the learned for centuries.

– George Lyman Kittredge, *The Old Farmer and His Almanack,* **1920**

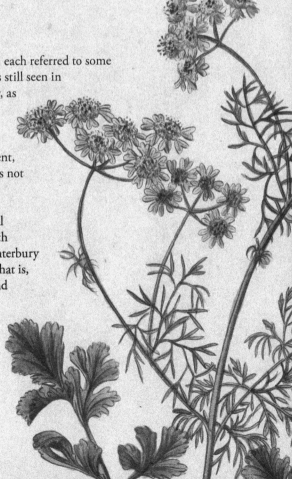

HISTORY OF HERBS IN
MEDICINE & MAGIC

The astrologian goes a step further than the herbalist, however, and insists that the other part of this knowledge should be regarded. To gain the utmost benefit from a herbal treatment it should be applied at an hour when the planet associated with the herb is active:

THE SUN: Almond, angelica, camomile, eye-bright, heart trefoil, juniper, mustard, rosemary, rue, saffron, sundew, vine and walnut.

THE MOON: Adder's-tongue, cabbage, cucumber, cress, lettuce, mouse-ear, orpine, pumpkin, saxifrage, trefoil.

MERCURY: Calamint, carraway, carrots, dill, endive, hazelnut, horehound, lavender, liquorice, mulberry, oats, parsley, wild carrots.

VENUS: Artichokes, beans, cherries, chestnut, elder, figwort, gooseberry, kidney-wort, marshmallow, mint, peppermint, raspberries, strawberries, wheat.

MARS: Aloes, barberry, cresses, catmint, hawkweed, garlic, honeysuckle, hops, horse-radish, leeks, mustard, onions, rhubarb, tobacco, wormwood.

JUPITER: Aniseed, apricot, asparagus, beetroot, endive, fig, hyssop, liverwort, lungwort, sage.

SATURN: Barley, comfrey, crosswort, heartsease, hemp, henbane, quince, rye, shepherd's-purse, spleenwort, thistle.

– **Edward Lyndoe,** *Everybody's Book of Fate and Fortune,* **1937**

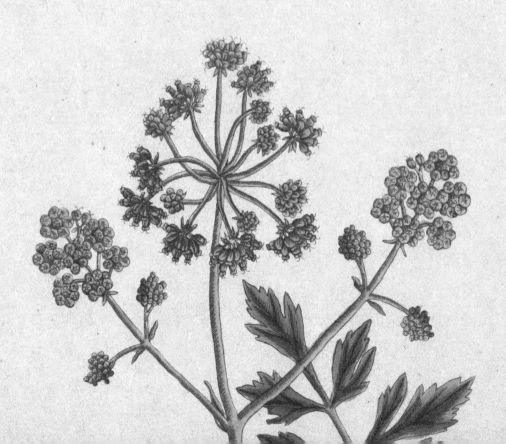

THE HERB GARDEN

In March and in April, from morning to night,
  in sowing and setting, good housewives delight;
To have in a garden or other like plot,
  to trim up their house, and to furnish their pot.

The nature of flowers, dame Physic doth shew;
  she teacheth them all, to be known to a few,
To set or to sow, or else sown to remove,
  how that should be practised, pain if ye love.

(...)

Time and ages, to sow or to gather be bold,
  but set to remove, when the weather is cold.
Cut all thing or gather, the moon in the wane,
  but sow in encreasing or give it his bane.

Now sets do ask watering, with pot or with dish,
  new sown do not so, if ye do as I wish:
Through cunning with dibble, rake, mattock and spade,
  by line, and by level, the garden is made.

Who soweth too lateward, hath seldom good seed,
  who soweth too soon little better shall speed,
Apt time and the season, so diverse to hit,
  layer and layer, help practice and wit.

     – Thomas Tusser, 'Marches Husbandrie', 1812

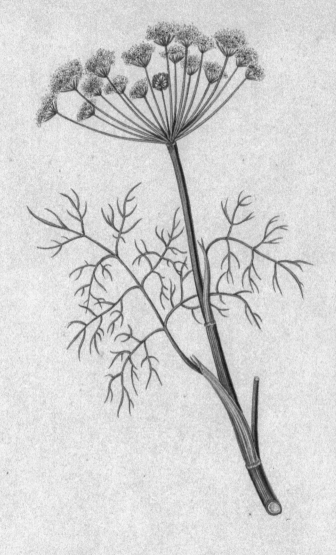

Garden.—To dream you are walking in a garden, is of a very favourable nature. It portends elevation in fortune and dignity. To the lover, it denotes great success and an advantageous marriage. To the tradesman, it promises increase of business. To the farmer, plentiful crops, and to the sailor, prosperous voyages.

     – Anon, *A Guide to Fortune Telling by Dreams*, 1894

Another name for the herb garden was the olitory; and the word herber, or herbar, would at first sight appear to be an herbarium, an herb garden.

     – Alice Morse Earle, *Old Time Gardens*, 1901

THE HERB GARDEN

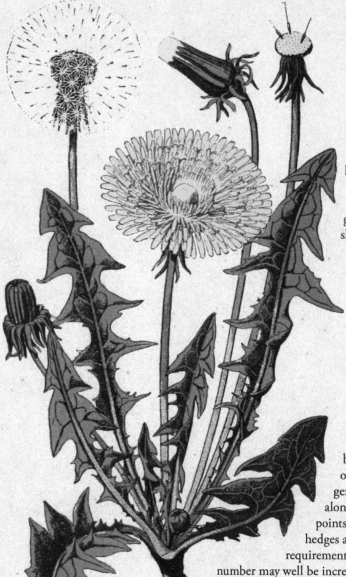

IN the days of our ancestors, the herb garden was a large and highly appreciated portion of the kitchen garden proper, and its entire planting and superintendence were the special work of the housewife. In it she grew herbs and simples, which were to give flavour to her dainty dishes or cure the small ailments of her household.

(...)

In every kitchen garden a sufficiently large piece of ground, according to the requirements of the family, should be devoted to the cultivation of sweet herbs.

(...)

The value of pot-herbs for culinary purposes, especially during the cold days of winter and early spring, is so great, that no house with a garden—even though it be a small one—should ever be without a ready and sufficient supply.

– **Tom Jerrold,** *Our War-Time Kitchen Garden: The Plants We Grow and How We Cook Them,* **1917**

The prettiest adjunct to a kitchen garden is the herb garden. It may be situated in one of the angles in order to take advantage of the walls as part of a formal boundary, and for shelter. Or it may lie on either side of the principal entrance, forming a small episode in the general scheme. A herb garden is attractive by its contents alone, and the necessity of having every plant accessible points to small beds and paths. Lavender and rosemary hedges are naturally associated with herbs, and though modern requirements call for less variety than in medieval times, the number may well be increased beyond kitchen needs for the sake of their beauty and fragrance.

– **Madeline Agar,** *Garden Design in Theory and Practice,* **1912**

Do you know what the scent of cut herbs is like on a hot summer day, with sweet peas in the background? In this herb garden there is sage, with its lovely blue flowers, lemon thyme, silver thyme, savory, hyssop, lavender, rosemary, rue, balm, marjoram, black peppermint, spearmint and parsley.

In this bed also grows the old-time bergamot, with its heavily-scented leaves and lovely tufts of crimson flowers.

– **Flora Klickmann,** *The Flower-Patch Among the Hills,* **1918**

THE HERB GARDEN

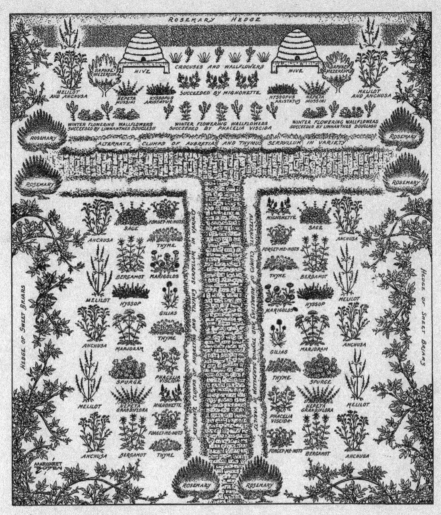

– Eleanour Sinclair Rohde, 'The Making of the Bee Garden', *The Times*, 1939

Propagation & Cultivation

Most herbs may be readily propagated by means of seeds. Some, however, such as tarragon, which does not produce seed, and several other perennial kinds, are propagated by division, layers, or cuttings. In general, propagation by means of seed is considered most satisfactory. Since the seeds in many instances are small or are slow to germinate, they are usually sown in shallow boxes or seed pans. When the seedlings are large enough to be handled they are transplanted to small pots or somewhat deeper flats or boxes, a couple of inches being allowed between the plants. When conditions are favorable in the garden; that is, when the soil is moist and warm and the season has become settled, the plantlets may be removed to permanent quarters.

THE HERB GARDEN

If the seed be sown out of doors, it is a good practice to sow a few radish seeds in the same row with the herb seeds, particularly if these latter take a long time to germinate or are very small, as marjoram, savory and thyme. The variety of radish chosen should be a turnip-rooted sort of exceedingly rapid growth, and with few and small leaves. The radishes serve to mark the rows and thus enable cultivation to commence much earlier than if the herbs were sown alone. They should be pulled early—the earlier the better after the herb plantlets appear. Never should the radishes be allowed to crowd the herbs.

In general, the most favorable exposure for an herb garden is toward the south, but lacking such an exposure should not deter one from planting herbs on a northern slope if this be the only site available. Indeed, such sites often prove remarkably good if other conditions are propitious and proper attention is given the plants. Similarly, a smooth, gently sloping surface is especially desirable, but even in gardens in which the ground is almost billowy the gardener may often take advantage of the irregularities by planting the moisture-loving plants in the hollows and those that like dry situations upon the ridges. Nothing like turning disadvantages to account!

No matter what the nature of the surface and the exposure, it is always advisable to give the herbs the most sunny spots in the garden, places where shade from trees, barns, other buildings and from fences cannot reach them. This is suggested because the development of the oils, upon which the flavoring of most of the herbs mainly depends, is best in full sunshine and the plants have more substance than when grown in the shade.

– **Eleanour Sinclair Rohde,** *The Old English Herbals,* **1922**

The ground should be dug over to about one foot in depth, and if such available, a thin layer of manure should be spread over the ground at this depth. The soil must be well broken up, and not left in lumps, particular care being taken with the surface, which should be pulverised with a rake or even passed through a coarse sieve, and then mixed with some silver sand.

– *Every Woman's Encyclopaedia Vol II,* **1800**

As to soil, a light, sandy loam, with a porous subsoil ensuring good drainage, will be the most favourable, as it is warmed quickly and is easily worked. A clay loam is less desirable as it cannot be worked so early in the season or after a spell of rain, and a very sandy soil is too porous and apt to scorch the plants. Good cultivation will, however, do much to remedy original defects in the soil.

For obtaining the best results in aromatic herbs a very rich soil is not required, as in such soils the growth is apt to be too rank, the quantity of volatile oil being small in proportion to the leafage produced.

– **Maurice Grenville Kains,** *Culinary Herbs,* **1912**

THE HERB GARDEN

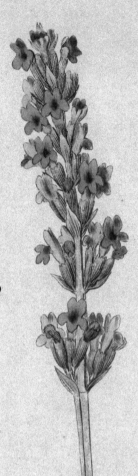

The Proper Method of Watering Gardens

The proper times for watering are the morning and the evening, to prevent the water from being heated by the sun; with the sole exception, however, of ocimum [basil], which requires to be watered at midday; indeed, this plant, it is generally thought, will grow with additional rapidity, if it is watered with boiling water when sown. All plants, when transplanted, grow all the better and larger for it, leeks and turnips more particularly. Transplanting, too, is attended with certain remedial effects, and acts as a preservative to certain plants, such as scallions, for instance, leeks, radishes, parsley, lettuces, rape, and cucumbers. All the wild plants are generally smaller in the leaf and stalk than the cultivated ones, and have more acrid juices, cunila [dittany], wild marjoram, and rue, for example.

— **Elder Pliny,** *The Natural History of Pliny,* c. 77 AD

Growing by the Moon

The moon, as everybody knows, was formerly thought to have a constant and powerful effect on men and things. This article of faith was universal and there is no occasion to dwell upon its antiquity. It has left plain traces upon our language in *moon-calf* for "monster", *moonstruck,* and *mooning,* as well as lunatic. As Othello Said

It is the very error of the moon:
She comes more near the earth than she was wont,
And makes men mad.

In the seventeenth and eighteenth centuries the influence of the moon on animal and vegetable life was not merely an article of faith among the ignorant. It was an accepted tenet of science.

— **George Lyman Kittredge,** *The Old Farmer and His Almanack,* 1920

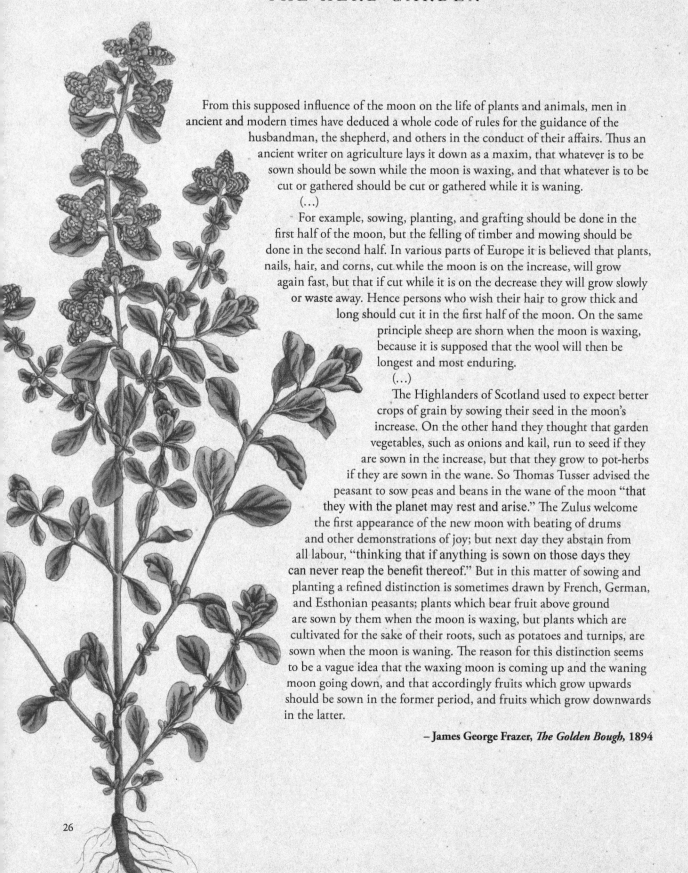

THE HERB GARDEN

From this supposed influence of the moon on the life of plants and animals, men in ancient and modern times have deduced a whole code of rules for the guidance of the husbandman, the shepherd, and others in the conduct of their affairs. Thus an ancient writer on agriculture lays it down as a maxim, that whatever is to be sown should be sown while the moon is waxing, and that whatever is to be cut or gathered should be cut or gathered while it is waning.

(...)

For example, sowing, planting, and grafting should be done in the first half of the moon, but the felling of timber and mowing should be done in the second half. In various parts of Europe it is believed that plants, nails, hair, and corns, cut while the moon is on the increase, will grow again fast, but that if cut while it is on the decrease they will grow slowly or waste away. Hence persons who wish their hair to grow thick and long should cut it in the first half of the moon. On the same principle sheep are shorn when the moon is waxing, because it is supposed that the wool will then be longest and most enduring.

(...)

The Highlanders of Scotland used to expect better crops of grain by sowing their seed in the moon's increase. On the other hand they thought that garden vegetables, such as onions and kail, run to seed if they are sown in the increase, but that they grow to pot-herbs if they are sown in the wane. So Thomas Tusser advised the peasant to sow peas and beans in the wane of the moon "that they with the planet may rest and arise." The Zulus welcome the first appearance of the new moon with beating of drums and other demonstrations of joy; but next day they abstain from all labour, "thinking that if anything is sown on those days they can never reap the benefit thereof." But in this matter of sowing and planting a refined distinction is sometimes drawn by French, German, and Esthonian peasants; plants which bear fruit above ground are sown by them when the moon is waxing, but plants which are cultivated for the sake of their roots, such as potatoes and turnips, are sown when the moon is waning. The reason for this distinction seems to be a vague idea that the waxing moon is coming up and the waning moon going down, and that accordingly fruits which grow upwards should be sown in the former period, and fruits which grow downwards in the latter.

– James George Frazer, *The Golden Bough*, 1894

26

PICKING, DRYING, AND STORING

Picking Ceremonies

Some of the most remarkable passages in the manuscripts are those concerning the ceremonies to be observed both in the picking and in the administering of herbs. What the mystery of plant life which has so deeply affected the minds of men in all ages and of all civilisations meant to our ancestors, we can but dimly apprehend as we study these ceremonies. They carry us back to that worship of earth and the forces of Nature which prevailed when Woden* was yet unborn. (…) It is to this age that the ceremonies in the picking of the herbs transport us, to the mystery of the virtues of herbs, the fertility of earth, the never-ceasing conflict between the beneficent forces of sun and summer and the evil powers of the long, dark northern winters. Closely intertwined with Nature worship we find the later Christian rites and ceremonies. For the new teaching did not oust the old, and for many centuries the mind of the average man halted half-way between the two faiths. If he accepted Christ he did not cease to fear the great hierarchy of unseen powers of Nature, the worship of which was bred in his very bone (…) The devil became one with the gloomy and terrible in Nature, with the malignant elves and dwarfs. Even with the warfare between the beneficent powers of sun and the fertility of Nature and the malignant powers of winter, the devil became associated. Nor did men cease to believe in the Wyrd, that dark, ultimate fate goddess who, though obscure, lies at the back of all Saxon belief. It was in vain that the Church preached against superstitions. Egbert, Archbishop of York, in his Penitential, strictly forbade the gathering of herbs with incantations and enjoined the use of Christian rites, but it is probable that even when these manuscripts were written, the majority at least of the common folk in these islands, though nominally Christian, had not deserted their ancient ways of thought. When the Saxon peasant went to gather his healing herbs he may have used Christian prayers and ceremonies, but he did not forget the goddess of the dawn. It is noteworthy how frequently we find the injunction that the herbs must be picked at sunrise or when day and night divide, how often stress is laid upon looking towards the east, and turning "as the sun goeth from east to south and west." In many there is the instruction that the herb is to be gathered "without use of iron" or "with gold and with hart's horn" (emblems of the sun's rays)… In some cases the herbs are to be gathered in silence, in others the man who gathers them is not to look behind him—a prohibition which occurs frequently in ancient superstitions. The ceremonies are all mysterious and suggestive, but behind them always lies the ancient ineradicable worship of Nature.

– Eleanour Sinclair Rohde, *The Old English Herbals*, 1922

*Or, Odin: Chief God of Germanic mythology

All herbs pulled on May Day Eve have a sacred healing power, if pulled in the name of the Holy Trinity; but if in the name of Satan, they work evil. Some herbs are malific if broken by the hand. So the plant is tied to a dog's foot, and when he runs it breaks, without a hand touching it, and may be used with safety.

A man pulled a certain herb on May Eve to cure his son who was sick to death. The boy recovered, but disappeared and was never heard of after, and the father died that day year. He had broken the fatal herb with the hand and so the doom fell on him.

Another man did the like, and gave the herb to his son to eat, who immediately began to bark like a dog, and so continued till he died.

– **Jane Wilde,** *Ancient Legends, Mystic Charms and Superstitions of Ireland,* 1919

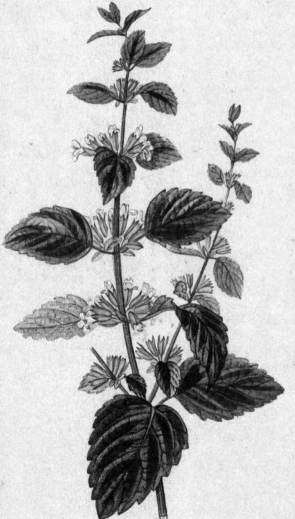

Picking & Gathering Herbs

Culinary herbs may be divided into three groups; those whose foliage furnishes the flavor, those whose seed is used and those few whose roots are prepared. In the kitchen, foliage herbs are employed either green or as decoctions or dried, each way with its special advocates, advantages and applications.

Green herbs, if freshly and properly gathered, are richest in flavoring substances and when added to sauces, fricassees, stews, etc., reveal their freshness by their particles as well as by their decidedly finer flavor. In salads they almost entirely supplant both the dried and the decocted herbs, since their fresh colors are pleasing to the eye and their crispness to the palate; whereas the specks of the dried herbs would be objectionable, and both these and the decoctions impart a somewhat inferior flavor to such dishes. Since herbs cannot, however, always be obtained throughout the year, unless they are grown in window boxes, they are infused or dried. Both infusing and drying are similar processes in themselves, but for best results they are dependent upon the observance of a few simple rules.

No matter in what condition or for what purpose they are to be used the flavors of foliage herbs are invariably best in well-developed leaves and shoots still in full vigor of growth. With respect to the plant as a whole, these flavors are most abundant and pleasant just before the flowers appear. And since they are generally due to essential oils, which are quickly dissipated by heat, they are more abundant in the morning than after the sun has reached the zenith. As a general rule, therefore, best results with foliage herbs, especially those to be used for drying and

infusing, may be secured when the plants
seem ready to flower, the harvest being
made as soon as the dew has dried and
before the day has become very warm.
The leaves of parsley, however, may be
gathered as soon as they attain that deep
green characteristic of the mature leaf; and
since the leaves are produced continuously for
many weeks, the mature ones may be removed
every week or so, a process which encourages the
further production of foliage and postpones the
appearance of the flowering stem.

To make good infusions the freshly gathered,
clean foliage should be liberally packed in stoppered
jars, covered with the choicest vinegar, and the jars kept
closed. In a week or two the fluid will be ready for use,
but in using it, trials must be made to ascertain its strength
and the quantity necessary to use. Usually only the clear
liquid is employed; sometimes, however, as with mint, the leaves
are very finely minced before being bottled and both liquid and
particles employed.

Tarragon, mint and the seed herbs, such as dill, are perhaps more
often used in ordinary cookery as infusions than otherwise.

– **Maurice Grenville Kains**, *Culinary Herbs*, 1912

In gathering herbs for medicinal purposes, we should not
only know the season when they should be culled, but we
should be qualified to comprehend the principles of which the
plant is composed
   – whether they be resins, alkaloids, or neutrals
   – and be able to also separate the one ingredient or element from
the other, as a distinct medicinal property, or combine the whole for the
purpose of a compound medical agent.

– **Nicholas Culpeper**, *Complete Herbal*, 1824

Gathering Leaves

Herbs ought to be gathered when the leaves have attained their full growth, though previously to the appearance of the flower-buds.

– Anon, Domestic Encyclopædia, 1802

Of leaves, choose only such as are green, and full of juice; pick them carefully, and reject decaying ones for they will putrify the rest, observed the places in which they grow best, and gather them there; for Betony in the shade is far better than that which grows in the sun, because it delights in the shade; also such herbs as grow well near water, should be gathered near it, though you may find some of them on dry ground.

The leaves of such herbs as run up to seed, are not so good when in flower as before; (some few excepted) if through negligence you have gathered them when in flower, take the tops and the flowers, rather than the leaf.

– Matthew Robinson, The New Family Herbal, 1863

Gathering Flowers

Flowers should be plucked on a clear day, when they are moderately expanded: after having been carefully selected, both herbs and flowers must be cautiously dried in a gentle heat, so that their strength and properties maybe more completely preserved: and, if they contain any subtle or volatile matter, it will be advisable to pulverize them as speedily as possible, and to keep such powder in closed glass vessels.

– Anon, Domestic Encyclopædia, 1802

Gathering Fruit

All fruits, however, should be allowed to become perfectly ripe, before they are removed from their stems or branches, excepting sloes, and one or two other astringents, that lose their virtues, if suffered to remain on the trees till they attain to maturity.

– Anon, Domestic Encyclopædia, 1802

Gathering Seeds

Nor should seeds be collected, until they
begin to grow dry, and are about to drop or shed
spontaneously; when they ought to be preserved
in an open situation, without being separated
from their husks; as these serve to protect them
from injuries of the air and weather.

– **Anon**, *Domestic Encyclopædia*, **1802**

The seed is that part of the plant which is endowed
with the vital faculty to bring forth its like, and it
contains potentially the whole plant in it. Gather them
in the place where they delight to grow. Let them be
full ripe when they are gathered. Dry them a little,
and but a little, in the sun before you lay them up. Keep
them in a dry place, they will keep many years; yet they are
best the first year; for they will grow soonest the first year after
being gathered, if sown; therefore being in their prime, they must
have more power.

– **Matthew Robinson**, *The New Family Herbal*, **1863**

Gathering Roots

Do not choose such as are rotten or worm-eaten,
but proper in their taste, colour and smell, such as
exceeded neither in softness nor hardness. The drier
the time you gather the roots, the better they are, having less
tendency to decay.

– **Matthew Robinson**, *The New Family Herbal*, **1863**

Gathering Bark

The barks of fruit are to be taken when the fruit is full ripe, as Oranges,
Lemons, &c. for then they come easier off; but the best way is to gather barks
only for present use.

– **Matthew Robinson**, *The New Family Herbal*, **1863**

Drying & Storing

When only a small quantity of an herb is to be dried, the old plan of hanging loose bunches from the ceiling of a warm, dry attic or a kitchen will answer. Better, perhaps, is the use of trays covered with clean, stout manilla paper upon which thin layers of the leaves are spread. These are placed either in hot sunlight or in the warm kitchen where warm air circulates freely. They must be turned once a day until all the moisture has been evaporated from the leaves and the softer, more delicate parts have become crisp. Then they may be crunched and crumbled between the hands, the stalks and the hard parts rejected and the powder placed in air-tight glass or earthenware jars or metal cans, and stored in a cool place. If there be the slightest trace of moisture in the powder, it should be still further dried to insure against mould. Prior to any drying process the cut leaves and stems should be thoroughly washed, to get rid of any trace of dirt. Before being dried as noted above, the water should all be allowed to evaporate. Evaporation may be hastened by exposing the herbs to a breeze in a shallow, loose basket, a wire tray or upon a table. While damp there is little danger of their being blown away. As they dry, however, the current of air should be more gentle.

The practice of storing powdered herbs in paper or pasteboard packages is bad, since the delicate oils readily diffuse through the paper and sooner or later the material becomes as valueless for flavoring purposes as ordinary hay or straw. This loss of flavor is particularly noticeable with sage, which is one of the easiest herbs to spoil by bad management.

– Maurice Grenville Kains, *Culinary Herbs***, 1912**

PICKING, DRYING, AND STORING

As these cannot always be procured green, it is convenient to have them in the house, dried and prepared, each in the proper season. The common method is to dry them in the sun, but their flavour is better preserved, by being put into a cool oven, or the meat screen, before a moderate fire, taking care not to scorch them. They should be gathered when just ripe, on a dry day. Cleanse them from dirt and dust, cut off the roots, put them before the fire, and dry them quickly, rather than by degrees. Pick off the leaves, pound and sift them; put the powder into bottles, and keep these closely stopped.

Basil, from the middle of August, to the same time in September.

Winter and Summer Savory, July and August.

Knotted Marjoram, July.

Thyme, Orange Thyme, and Lemon Thyme, June and July.

Mint, end of June and through July.

Sage, August and September.

Tarragon, June, July, and August.

Chervil, May, June, July.

Burnet, June, July, August.

Parsley, May, June, July.

Fennel, May, June, July.

Elder Flowers, May, June, July.

Orange Flowers, May, June, and July.

– Anne Cobbet, *The English Housekeeper,* **1851**

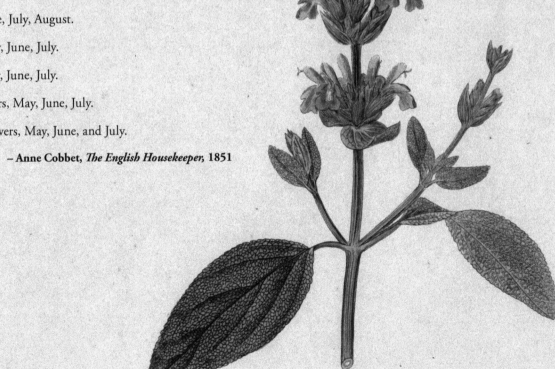

A TWELFTH-CENTURY PRAYER TO EARTH

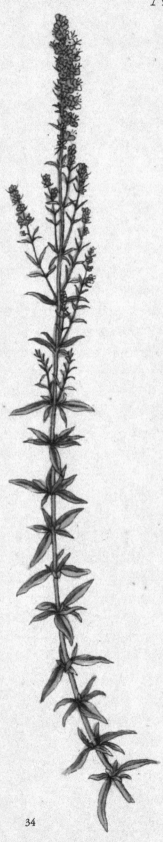

[It was] believed (…) that natural forces and natural objects were endued with mysterious powers whom it was necessary to propitiate by special prayers. Not only the stars of heaven, but springs of water and the simple wayside herbs, were to them directly associated with unseen beings. (…) Even in a twelfth-century herbal we find a prayer to Earth:

"Earth, divine goddess, Mother Nature who generatest all things and bringest forth anew the sun which thou hast given to the nations; Guardian of sky and sea and of all gods and powers and through thy power all nature falls silent and then sinks in sleep. And again thou bringest back the light and chasest away night and yet again thou coverest us most securely with thy shades. Thou dost contain chaos infinite, yea and winds and showers and storms; thou sendest them out when thou wilt and causest the seas to roar; thou chasest away the sun and arousest the storm. Again when thou wilt thou sendest forth the joyous day and givest the nourishment of life with thy eternal surety; and when the soul departs to thee we return. Thou indeed art duly called great Mother of the gods; thou conquerest by thy divine name. Thou art the source of the strength of nations and of gods, without thee nothing can be brought to perfection or be born; thou art great queen of the gods. Goddess! I adore thee as divine; I call upon thy name; be pleased to grant that which I ask thee, so shall I give thanks to thee, goddess, with one faith. "Hear, I beseech thee, and be favourable to my prayer. Whatsoever herb thy power dost produce, give, I pray, with goodwill to all nations to save them and grant me this my medicine. Come to me with thy powers, and howsoever I may use them may they have good success and to whomsoever I may give them. Whatever thou dost grant it may prosper. To thee all things return. Those who rightly receive these herbs from me, do thou make them whole. Goddess, I beseech thee; I pray thee as a suppliant that by thy majesty thou grant this to me.

"Now I make intercession to you all ye powers and herbs and to your majesty, ye whom Earth parent of all hath produced and given as a medicine of health to all nations and hath put majesty upon you, be, I pray you, the greatest help to the human race. This I pray and beseech from you, and be present here with your virtues, for she who created you hath herself promised that I may gather you into the goodwill of him on whom the art of medicine was bestowed, and grant for health's sake good medicine by grace of your powers. I pray grant me through your virtues that whatsoe'er is wrought by me through you may in all its powers have a good and speedy effect and good success and that I may always be permitted with the favour of your majesty to gather you into my hands and to glean your fruits. So shall I give thanks to you in the name of that majesty which ordained your birth."

– Translation from 'Early English Magic and Medicine by Dr. Charles Singer. Proceedings of the British Academy, Vol. IV.', Eleanour Sinclair Rohde, *The Old English Herbals*, 1922

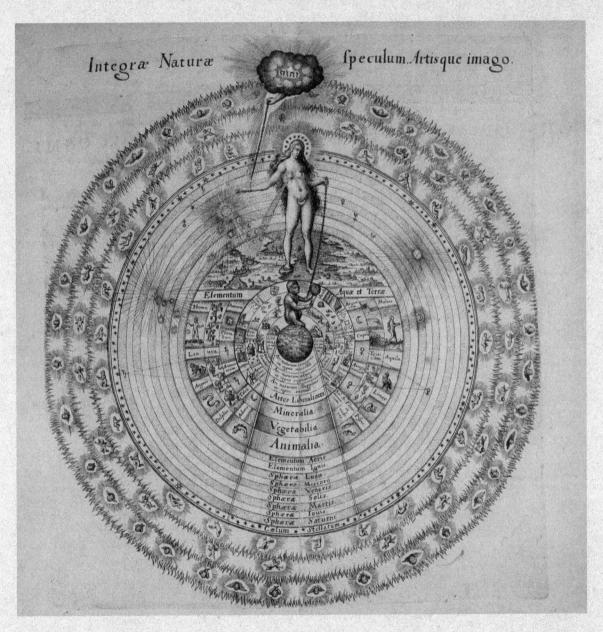

Robert Fludd, 'Integrae Naturae speculum Artisque imago' – The Mirror of the Whole of Nature and the Image of Art,
Utriusque cosmi maioris scilicet et minoris metaphysica, physica atque technica historia, 1617

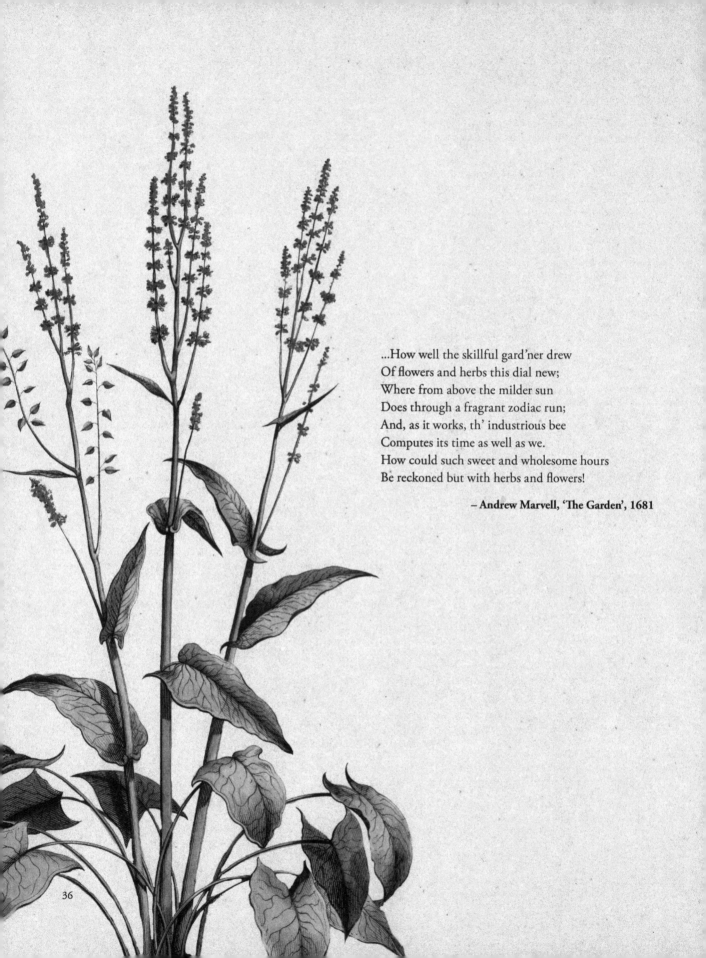

...How well the skillful gard'ner drew
Of flowers and herbs this dial new;
Where from above the milder sun
Does through a fragrant zodiac run;
And, as it works, th' industrious bee
Computes its time as well as we.
How could such sweet and wholesome hours
Be reckoned but with herbs and flowers!

— **Andrew Marvell, 'The Garden', 1681**

THE GROWER'S
HERB LIST

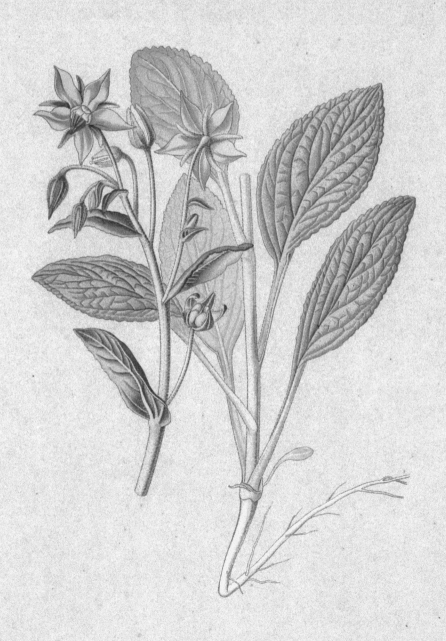

Speak not – whisper not;
Here bloweth thyme and bergamot;
Softly on the evening hour,
Secret herbs their spices shower.
Dark-spiked rosemary and myrrh,
Lean-stalked, purple lavender;
Hides within her bosom, too,
All her sorrows, bitter rue.

Breathe not – trespass not;
Of this green and darkling spot,
Latticed from the moon's beams;
Perchance a distant dreamer dreams;
Perchance upon its darkening air,
The unseen ghosts of children fare,
Faintly swinging, sway and sweep,
Like lovely sea-flowers in its deep;
While, unmoved, to watch and ward,
Amid its gloomed and daisied sward,
Stands with bowed and dewy head
That one little Leaden lad.

– Walter de la Mare, 'The Sunken Garden', 1917

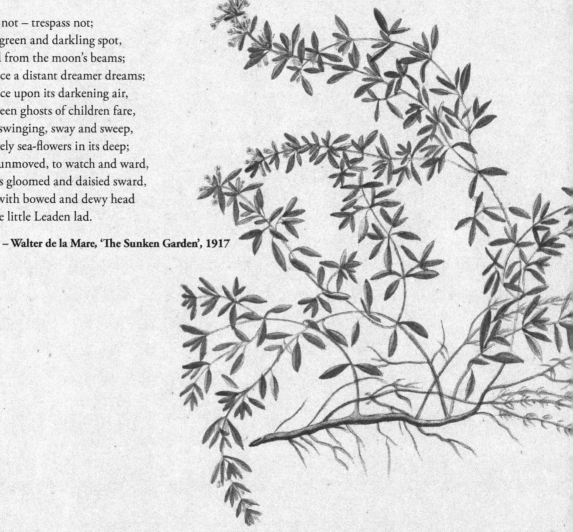

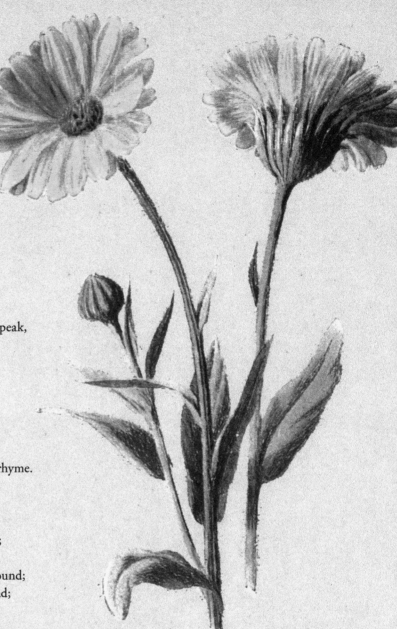

XI.

Herbs, too, she knew, and well of each could speak,
That in her garden sipp'd the silv'ry dew,
Wher no vain flower disclosed a gaudy streak;
But herbs for use, and physic, not a few,
Of grey renown, within those borders grew;
The tufted basil, pun-provoking thyme,
Fresh balm, and marygold of cheerful hue;
The lowly gill, that never dares to climb;
And more I fain would sing, disdaining here to rhyme.

XII.

Yet euphrasy may not be left unsung,
That gives dim eyes to wander leagues around;
And pungent radish, biting infant's tongue;
And plantain ribb'd, that heals the reaper's wound;
And marjoram sweet, in shepherd's posie found;
And lavender, whose pikes of azure bloom
Shall be, erewhile, in arid bundles bound,
To lurk amidst the labours of her loom,
And crown her kerchiefs clean with mickle rare perfume.

– William Shenstone, 'The School Mistress', 1782

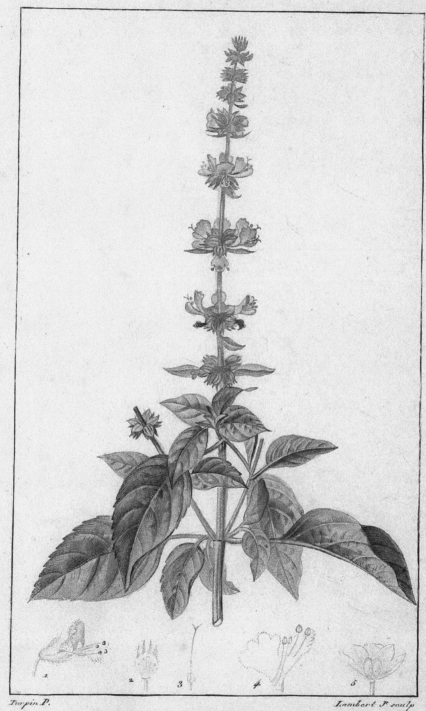

Turpin P.

Lambert F. sculp

BASILIC.

a.l.l.

BASIL

Other Names: Sweet Basil
Latin Name: Ocimum basilicum
Symbolises: Hatred
Type: Annual, not hardy
Natural Habitat: India
Growing Zone: 10–11
Site: Full sun in well-drained soil. Grows well in containers
Sow: March to June. Successional plantings for longer cropping
Harvest: May to October. Six to eight weeks from sowing
Usable Parts: Leaves
Companion Plants: Oregano, parsley, tomatoes, peppers, and lettuce
Herbal Astrology: Mars

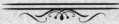

A culinary herb beloved by the masses, basil's fragrant leaves are a revered ingredient in kitchens. Its uses in modern cookery often overshadow its mythical past. It was once believed to hold magical properties, becoming a common ingredient in love spells. John Keats pays homage to this association with love in his famous poem 'Isabella', a beautiful narrative tale where a basil plant comes to represent the undying affection between young lovers struck by tragedy.

The greater of Ordinary Basil rises up usually with one upright stalk, diversly branching forth on all sides, with two leaves at every joint, which are somewhat broad and round, yet pointed, of a pale green colour, but fresh; a little snipped about the edges, and of a strong healthy scent. The flowers are small and white, and standing at the tops of the branches, with two small leaves at the joints, in some places green, in others brown, after which come black seed. The root perishes at the approach of Winter, and therefore must be new sown every year.

– Nicholas Culpeper, *Complete Herbal,* 1824

BASIL

continued.

Fine basil desireth it may be her lot,
To grow as the andfulwer, trim in a pot;
That ladies and gentles to whom ye do serve
May help her, as needeth, poor life to preserve.

– Thomas Tusser, *Five Hundred Pointes*
of Good Husbandry, **1812**

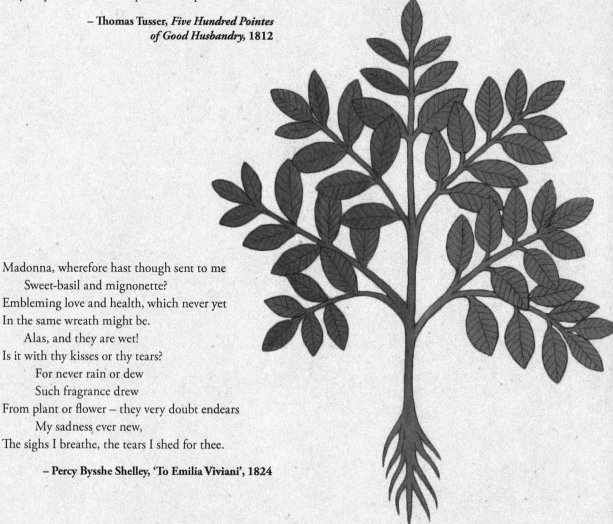

Madonna, wherefore hast though sent to me
   Sweet-basil and mignonette?
Embleming love and health, which never yet
In the same wreath might be.
   Alas, and they are wet!
Is it with thy kisses or thy tears?
    For never rain or dew
    Such fragrance drew
From plant or flower – they very doubt endears
    My sadness ever new,
The sighs I breathe, the tears I shed for thee.

– Percy Bysshe Shelley, 'To Emilia Viviani', 1824

BASIL

continued.

In the Garden

It is a tender annual, delicately aromatic, and should be used green to be of its best. Coming originally from India, it is usually first raised in a hot-bed, and the plants are pricked out at the end of June.

– Isabella Beeton, *Gardening,* **1861**

They are best raised under glass in March or early May and planted out nine inches apart in mid-May.

– Eleanour Sinclair Rohde, *Herbs and Herb Gardening,* **1936**

Most people stroake Garden Basil, which leaves a grateful Smell on the Hand; and he will have it, that such stroaking from a fair lady preserves the life of the Basil.

– Thomas Tusser, *Five Hundred Pointes of Good Husbandry,* **1812**

In the Kitchen

Basil vinegar is made by steeping the leaves in vinegar, and is used for flavouring when the fresh plant cannot be procured.

– Charles Herman Senn, *A Pocket Dictionary of Foods & Culinary Encyclopaedia,* **1908**

A modern gardener writes that sweet basil has the flavour of cloves, that it is always demanded by French cooks, and that it is much used to flavour soups, and occasionally salads. M. de la Quintinye, director of the gardens of Louis XIV., shows that over two hundred years ago French cooks were of the same mind about basil as they are today; besides mentioning it for the uses just named, he adds, "it is likewise used in ragouts, especially dry ones, for which reason we take care to keep some for winter."

– Rosalind Northcote, *The Book of Herbs,* **1903**

The seeds and stems are dried and used for flavoring soups and sauces, etc. It is also used when young and tender to mix with cooked vegetable salads, such as potatoes, beets, peas, beans, etc.

– Jules Arthur Harder, *The Physiology of Taste,* **1885**

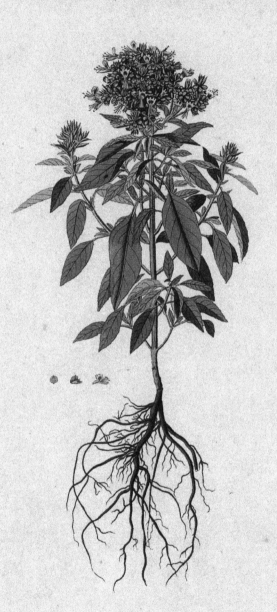

BASIL

ANCIENT KNOWLEDGE, VIRTUES, AND LORE

Medicinal Properties and Remedies

Being applied to the place bitten by venomous beasts, or stung by a wasp or hornet, it speedily draws the poison to it; Every like draws his like.

– Nicholas Culpeper, *Complete Herbal,* 1824

It may be eaten by Women to dry up their milk: or if upon tryal they find any inconveniency of taking it this way, it may be applyed to the breasts outwardly being first bruised a little.
(…)

The seeds are used to help the trembling of the heart and to comfort the same, as also to expel Melancholy or sadnesse.
(…)

Mixed with honey and used, it taketh a way spots in the face.

–William Coles, *Adam in Eden; Or, Natures Paradise,* 1657

Herbal Magic

If two leaves of basil are placed upon a hot coal and burn away quietly, the marriage will be a happy one; but if they crackle to a certain extent, the lives of the couple, who are represented by the two leaves, will be ruffled by quarrels. If, however, the leaves crackle very much and fall apart, it shows such incompatibility of temper that the parties interested will be wise if they decide to separate before being bound by the marriage tie.

–Winifred S. Blackman, *The Magical and Ceremonial Uses of Fire,* 1916

If a girl gives a man a present with a sprig of basil hidden in it so that he takes the gift without knowing anything about the basil, his love will be hers.

– Diana Hawthorne, *Laurie's Complete Fortune Teller,* 1946

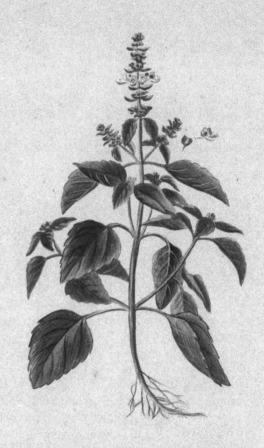

Folk Beliefs

The derivation of the name Basil is uncertain. Some authorities say it comes from the Greek basileus, a king, because, as Parkinson says, 'the smell thereof is so excellent that it is fit for a king's house,' or it may have been termed royal, because it was used in some regal unguent or medicine. One rather unlikely theory is that it is shortened from basilisk, a fabulous creature that could kill with a look. This theory may be based on a strange old superstition that connected the plant with scorpions. Parkinson tells us that 'being gently handled it gave a pleasant smell but being hardly wrung and bruised would breed scorpions. It is also observed that scorpions doe much rest and abide under these pots and vessells wherein Basil is planted.'

It was generally believed that if a sprig of Basil were left under a pot it would in time turn to a scorpion. Superstition went so far as to affirm that even smelling the plant might bring a scorpion into the brain.

– Maude Grieve, *A Modern Herbal,* **1931**

In India, where the basil is native, it is a holy herb, dedicated to Vishnu, whose wife, Lakshmi, it is in disguise. To break a sprig of the plant fills him with pain, and he commonly denies the prayers of such as trespass against it; yet it is permitted to wear the seeds as a rosary and to remove a leaf, for every good Hindu goes to his rest with a basil leaf on his breast, which he has only to show at the gate of heaven to be admitted. In Persia and Malaysia basil is planted on graves while in Egypt women scatter the flowers on the resting places of their dead. These faiths and observances are out of keeping with the Greek idea that it represented hate and misfortune, and they painted poverty, in apotheosis, as a ragged woman with a basil at her side.

In Romania, the maid who has set her cap for a young man will surely win his affection if she can get him to accept a sprig of basil from her hand. In Moldavia, too, if he so accept it, his wanderings cease from that hour, and he is hopelessly hers. In Crete, where it is cultivated as a house plant, it symbolizes "love washed with tears," but in parts of Italy it is a love-token, and goes by the name of little-love and kiss-me-Nicholas, a name that of course invites the swain when he discovers it in the hand or in the hair of his mistress.

– Charles Montgomery Skinner, *Myths and Legends of Flowers, Fruits and Plants,* **1911**

45

BASIL

Isabella, or, The Pot of Basil

In a worthy tribute to the popular herb, Keats' narrative poem, 'Isabella; or, The Pot of Basil' (1818), is a sweet tale of heartbreak and courage in the face of tragedy. Keats borrowed the tale from a story in Boccaccio's The Decameron *(1620). While the plant keeps its sinister associations with jealousy and crime – said to have come from an ancient Greek tradition where basil symbolises hatred and despair – in Keats' poem, the herb transforms into a symbol of undying love, even after death.*

Consumed by grief after her beloved Lorenzo is murdered by her brothers due to their secret love affair, Isabella refuses to accept his death. She steals away, removing his head from his corpse, and plants it in a pot of basil. Tending to the plant daily, the adoration for her lost love strengthens, and as time passes, the plant grows strong. Isabella spends her days watering the basil with her tears and eventually dies of a broken heart. Her thriving basil plant symbolises her enduring love for her beloved.

Isabella, whose story has been told by Boccaccio, Keats, and Hunt, in tale, poem, and picture, was a maid of Messina who, left to her own resources by her brothers—they being rich and absorbed in business—found solace in the company of Lorenzo, the comely manager of their enterprises. The brothers noted the meetings, but, wishing to avoid a scandal, they pretended to have seen nothing. Finally they bade Lorenzo to a festival outside of the city, and there slew him. They told their sister that Lorenzo had been sent on a long journey, but when days, weeks, even months, had passed, she could no longer restrain her uneasiness, and asked when he would return. "What do you mean?" demanded one of the brothers. "What have you in common with such as Lorenzo? Ask for him farther, and you shall be answered as you deserve."

Isabella kept her chamber for that day, a victim to fears and doubts; but in her solitude she called on her lover, making piteous moan that he would return. And he did so; for when she had fallen asleep, Lorenzo's ghost appeared, pale, blood-drabbled, with garments rent and mouldy, and addressed her: "Isabella, I can never return to you, for on the day we saw each other last your brothers slew me."

After telling where she might find his body, the speaker melted into air, and in fright she awoke. Unable to shake off the impression of the scene, she fled to the scene of the tragedy, and there, in a space of ground recently disturbed, she came upon Lorenzo, lying as in sleep, for there was a preserving virtue in the soil. She was first for moving the corpse to holy ground, but this would invite discovery, so with a knife she removed the head, and, borrowing "a great and goodly pot," laid it therein, folded in a fair linen cloth, and covered it with earth. Some basil of Salerno she then planted, and it was her comfort to guard the growing plant sprung from her lover's flesh, and water it with essences and orange water, but oftener with tears. Tended so with love and care, the plant grew strong and filled the room with sweetness. Her home-staying and the pallor of weeping led the brothers to wonder, and, thinking to cure her of a mental malady, they took away the flower. She cried unceasingly for its return, and the men, still marvelling, spilt it from its tub to find if she had hidden anything beneath its root; and in truth she had, for there they found the mouldering head which, by its fair and curling hair, they recognized as Lorenzo's. Realizing that the murder had been discovered, they buried the relic anew, and fled to Naples. Isabella died of heart-emptiness, still lamenting her pot of basil.

– Charles Montgomery Skinner, *Myths and Legends of Flowers, Fruits and Plants*, 1911

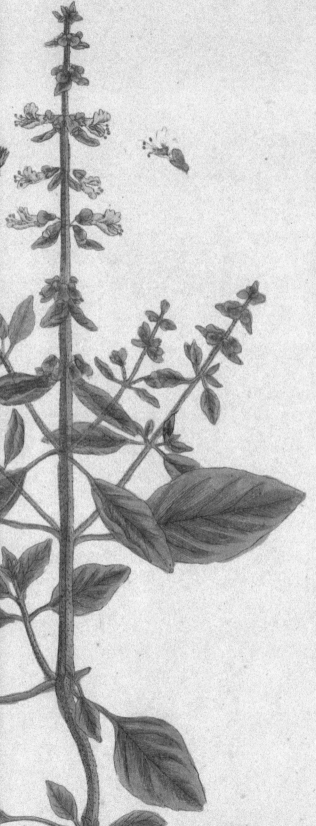

BASIL

continued.

LII.

Then in a silken scarf, - sweet with the dews
    Of precious flowers pluck'd in Araby,
And divine liquids come with odorous ooze
    Through the cold serpent pipe refreshfully, -
She wrapp'd it up; and for its tomb did choose
    A garden-pot, wherein she laid it by,
And cover'd it with mould, and o'er it set
Sweet Basil, which her tears kept ever wet.

LIII.

And she forgot the stars, the moon, and sun,
    And she forgot the blue above the trees,
And she forgot the dells where waters run,
    And she forgot the chilly autumn breeze;
She had no knowledge when the day was done,
    And the new morn she saw not: but in peace
Hung over her sweet Basil evermore,
And moisten'd it with tears unto the core.

LIV.

And so she ever fed it with thin tears,
    Whence thick, and green, and beautiful it grew,
So that it smelt more balmy than its peers
    Of Basil-tufts in Florence; for it drew
Nurture besides, and life, from human fears,
    From the fast mouldering head there shut from view:
So that the jewel, safely casketed,
Came forth, and in perfumed leafits spread.

– **John Keats, extract from 'Isabella, or, The
Pot of Basil', 1818**

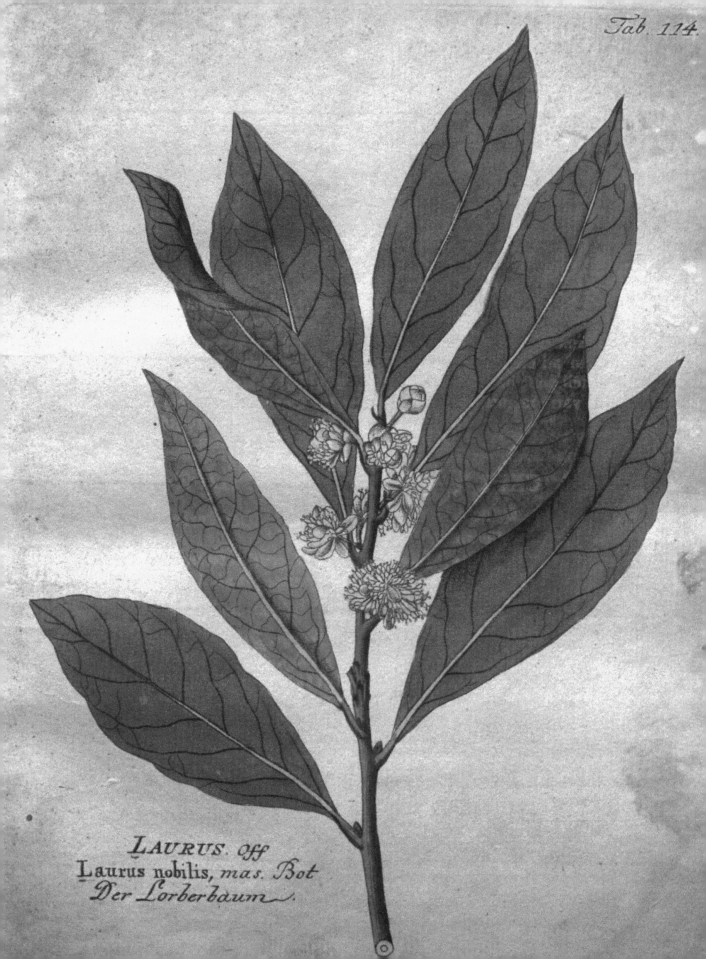

Tab. 114.

LAURUS. off
Laurus nobilis, mas. Bot
Der Lorberbaum.

BAY

continued.

Other Names: Sweet Bay, Noble Laurel, Roman Laurel
Latin Name: Laurus nobilis
Symbolises: Glory, I change but in death
Laurel—content, success, marriage
Laurel (to pick it)—triumph
Laurel (to be crowned with it)—vanity
Type: Half-hardy shrub or small tree
Natural Habitat: India
Growing Zone: 8–10
Site: Full sun to light shade. Fertile, well-drained soil, or high quality potting compost. Suitable for containers
Sow: Start with a purchased plant, or take cuttings March to June
Harvest: All year round
Usable Parts: Leaves and branches
Companion Plants: Parsley, rosemary, sage, and thyme
Herbal Astrology: The Sun

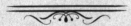

The bay tree can be grown in any garden, with its structural stature providing ornamental and fruitful bounty for the kitchen. The berries, not often employed these days, were believed by herbalists such as Nicholas Culpeper to be a heal-all for bruises and cuts when mixed into an oil. Another herb commonly used in cooking, its leaves are often used to flavour soups, stews, and sauces.

The Bay or Laurell tree commeth oftentimes to the height of a tree of a mean bigness: it is full of boughes, covered with a green barke: the leaves thereof are long, broad, hard, of colour green, sweetly smelling, and in taste somewhat bitter. The flowers alongst the boughes and leaves are of a green colour, the berries are more long than round, and be covered with a blacke rinde or pill: the kernel within is cloven into two parts like that of the Peach and almond, and other such, of a brown yellowish colour, sweet of smell, in taste somewhat bitter, with a little sharp or biting qualitie.

– John Gerard, *The Herball, or, Generall Historie of Plantes,* **1597**

BAY

continued.

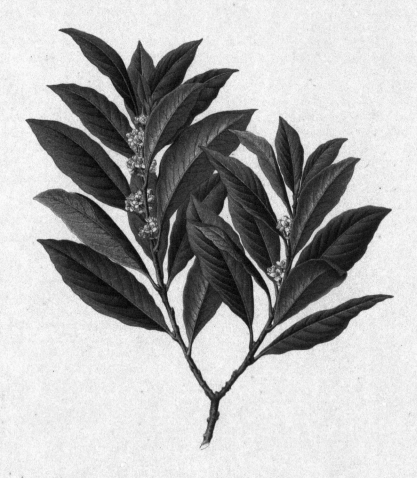

Then in my lavender I'll lay,
Muscado put among it,
And here and there a leaf of bay,
Which still shall run along it.

– Michael Drayton, *Muses Elizium,* **1630**

'Tis thought the king is dead; we will not stay.
The bay trees in our country are all withered.

– William Shakespeare, *Richard II,* **Act 2, Scene 4, 1595**

In the Garden

Bay and box trees are expensive, but long-lived if given moderate care, and the white and pink oleanders which flower continually are also well worth a place on the terrace or in the garden. These three varieties need only to be kept clean, nourished, given enough water, not allowed to freeze, and occasionally re-tubbed.

When the tubs containing bay and box trees and oleanders are brought forth from their winter quarters, they require immediate attention. They should first be watered with a strong force to cleanse them thoroughly, and then looked over for scale, which should be carefully scraped away; if the bay trees have accumulated any black mildew, it can be scrubbed off with a nail-brush, which, although a long and slow process if the trees are large, is the only one which is effective. The trees should then be sprayed with a strong solution of Ivory soap, some of the earth removed from the top of the tubs, and some soot, which is the best fertilizer for bay and box trees, dug in about the roots, and the tub then filled up with cow manure.

– Helena Rutherford Ely, *The Practical Flower Garden*, **1913**

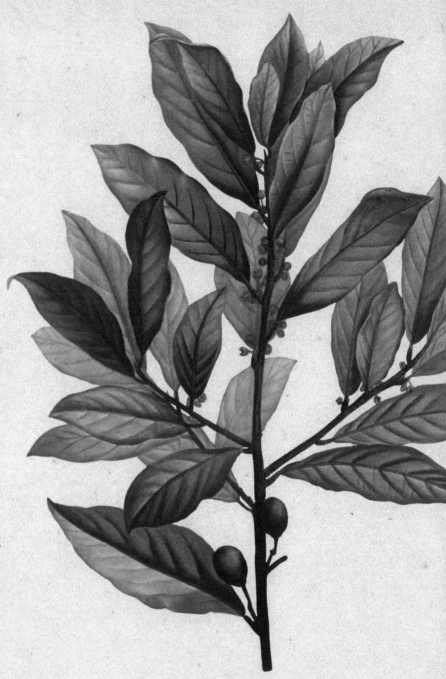

BAY

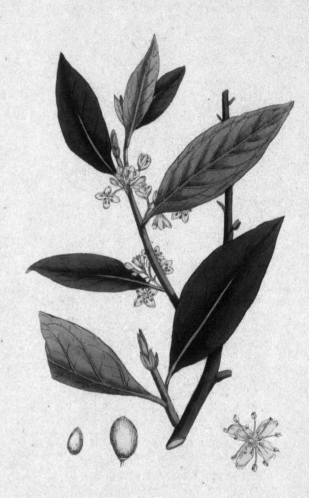

Prepare your wreaths, Aonian maids divine,
   To strew the tranquil bed where I shall sleep;
   In tears, the myrtle and the laurel steep,
And let Erato's hand the trophies twine.
No parian marble, there, with labour'd line,
   Shall bid the wand'ring lover stay to weep;
   There holy silence shall her vigils keep.
Save, when the nightingale such woes as mine
   Shall sadly sing; as twilight's curtains spread,
There shall the branching lotos widely wave,
   Sprinkling soft show'rs upon the lily's head,
Sweet drooping emblem for a lover's grave!
   And there shall Phaon pearls of pity shed,
To gem the vanquish'd heart he scorn'd to save!

          – Mary Robinson, 'To the Muses', 1796

In the Kitchen

   These leaves are much used for culinary purposes, being indispensable for stews, etc.. For these purposes they should be used in their dry state, as they then lose their bitter taste. In their green state they are used for pickling, and in imparting an aromatic taste to meats.

          – Jules Arthur Harder, *The Physiology of Taste*, 1885

BAY

continued.

ANCIENT KNOWLEDGE, VIRTUES, AND LORE

Medicinal Properties and Remedies

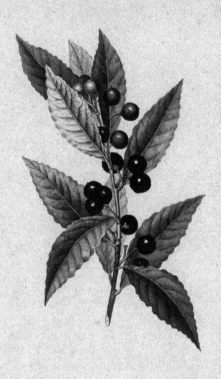

The berries are very effectual against all poison of venomous creatures, and the sting of wasps and bees; as also against the pestilence, or other infectious diseases, and therefore put into sundry treacles for that purpose (...) They wonderfully help all cold and rheumatic distillations from the brain to the eyes, lungs or other parts; and being made into an electuary with honey, do help the consumption, old coughs, shortness of breath, and thin rheums; as also the megrim.

The oil made of the berries is very comfortable in all cold griefs of the joints, nerves, arteries, stomach, belly, or womb, and helps palsies, convulsions, cramp, aches, tremblings, and numbness in any part, weariness also, and pains that come by sore travelling. All griefs and pains proceeding from wind, either in the head, stomach, back, belly, or womb, by anointing the parts affected therewith: And pains in the ears are also cured by dropping in some of the oil, or by receiving into the ears the fume of the decoction of the berries through a funnel. The oil takes away the marks of the skin and flesh by bruises, falls, &c. and dissolves the congealed blood in them. It helps also the itch, scabs, and weals in the skin.

– Nicholas Culpeper, *Complete Herbal*, 1824

A French apothecary has discovered an excellent and very cheap substitute for quinine, in powdered laurel-leaf. The leaves of the laurel (*Laurus nobilis*) are slowly dried over the fire in a close vessel, and then powdered. One gramme (15½ grains) is a dose, and is taken in a glass of cold water. The drug so taken produces no bad effects, and soon, it is said, breaks up the most obstinate intermittent fevers.

– *Popular Science Monthly*, Vol. III, 1873

To Help the Face with Red Pimples

Take Bay-berries, and pluck off the husks, and make a fine powder thereof, and temper it with honey: anoint your face therewith fix times, and it will help you.

– Hugh Plat, *Delights for Ladies to Adorn their Persons, Tables, Closets, and Distillatories*, 1644

BAY

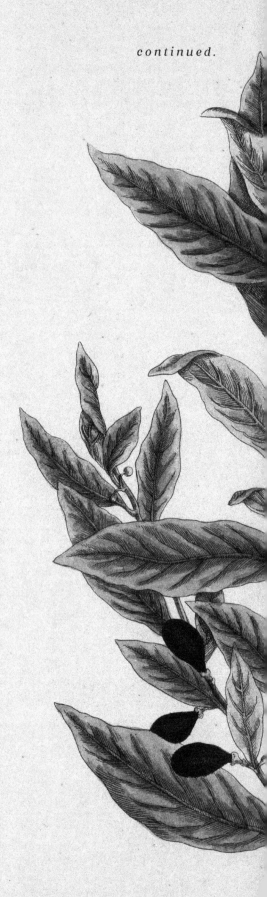

Herbal Magic

It is a tree of the sun, and under the celestial sign Leo, and resists the witchcraft very potently as also all the evils old Saturn can do the body of man, and they are not a few; for it is the speech of one and I am mistaken if it were not Mizaldus, that neither witch nor devil, thunder nor lightning will hurt a man where a Bay tree is.

> – **Nicholas Culpeper**, *Complete Herbal*, 1824

On the eve of Valentine's Day it was the custom for a man to get five bay leaves, pin four of them to the corners of his pillow and the fifth in the centre, and then go to sleep. If he dreamed of a girl, he would marry her before the year was out.

> – **Astra Cielo**, *Signs, Omens, and Superstitions*, 1918

Gather five leaves from a bay or laurel bush at the time of the full moon. One must be fastened to the middle of the pillow and one to each corner. That done, the girl must stand at the window, and raising her eyes to the moon, she must say aloud:

Sweetheart, come to me this night,
Riding on the moonbeams bright.
Be beside me in my sleep,
And thy thoughts on me do keep.

> – **Diana Hawthorne**, *Laurie's Complete Fortune Teller*, 1946

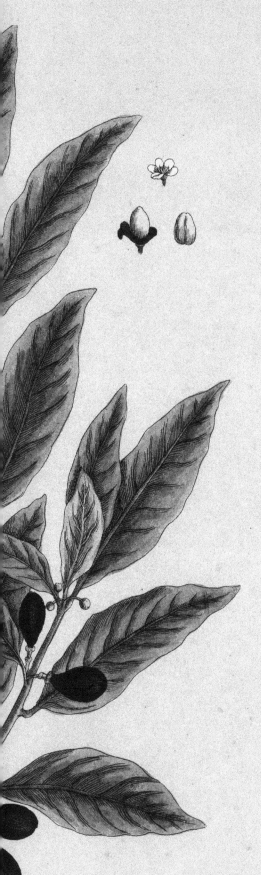

Folk Beliefs

The bay is an emblem of the resurrection, for, according to Sir Thomas Browne, when seemingly dead, it will revive from the root, and its dry leaves resume their wonted vitality.

— **Jane Wilde,** *Ancient Legends, Mystic Charms and Superstitions of Ireland,* **1919**

The Bible refers to the very ancient superstition that the flourishing of the bay tree meant good, and its withering, evil:
   "I have seen the wicked in great power, and spreading himself like a green bay tree.
   "Yet he passed away, and, lo, he was not: yea, I sought him, but he could not be found." *Psalms xxxvii. 35 and 36.*

— **Francis Bacon,** *The Essays of Francis Bacon,* **1908**

Laurel was prized by the Greeks as an averter of ill, and hung over their doors to keep off lightning. From a token of safety, it became a badge of victory. Generals sent dispatches to the emperor encased in laurel leaves. The leaves were woven into garlands and crowns for victors in the games, as were myrtle, olive, pine, and parsley. If laurel were put under a rhymester's pillow, they made a poet of him, and if he read his verses in a university he was crowned with the leaves and berries; so we have the word baccalaureate, which means, laurel berry; and as the student was supposed to keep so closely to his books that he had no thought for matrimony, the derivative word bachelor came to be applied to an unmarried man. Laurel also gave power to soothsayers to look into the future.

— **Charles Montgomery Skinner,** *Myths and Legends of Flowers, Trees, Fruits and Plants,* **1911**

BAY

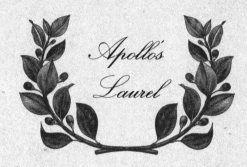

This transformative myth tells how Apollo pursued the wood nymph Daphne to be his wife. She evaded his advances, eventually shifting into a laurel tree to escape him. Despite her arboreous form, Apollo remained undeterred and devoted himself to her. In homage to their impossible romance, Apollo crowned himself with her leaves, coining them a sign of victory for any champion. He chose the laurel as his precious tree, vowing to honour her forever.

It was because of Apollo that Daphne was unhappy. Daphne was a wild, young thing. She loved the beasts and birds and flowers better than she did human companionship, and she wished for nothing better than to play among the forest trees all the rest of her life. But the River-god, her father, had told her that he wished her to marry Apollo, the golden-haired, young Sun-god. Apollo was as clever as he was fine-looking, for he could play on any kind of musical instrument that you might choose to give him, and speak in poetry as easily as he could in prose. But Daphne did not wish to marry anybody.

"Let me be free," she said, "to live among the trees and flowers as I have always done. Nothing else can ever make me happy—and I don't like Apollo, anyway."

But at this, her father only laughed and said: "Well, well, I am not going to make you marry anyone that you dislike, but, for all that, the day is coming when you will change your mind. You may like Apollo better by and by."

Daphne was not pleased to have her father laugh at her, and she did not wish to talk about Apollo. So she slipped away and ran off to the woods where she could forget all about the whole matter.

But it wasn't so easy to forget about Apollo, for he knew that Daphne loved to spend her time in the shady woods, and he had come there to find her. She was sitting on a mossy bank beside a little brook, when she looked up suddenly and saw Apollo coming toward her. Up she jumped from the ground and started to run away from him. Apollo saw that she was frightened, and called to her.

"Daphne, dear, don't run away; I want to talk to you. I wouldn't hurt you for the world. Don't be afraid of me."

But the sound of his voice lent wings to Daphne's feet. She ran as fast as she could go, and Apollo, not wishing to be left behind, ran after her. Now, though Daphne could run like a deer, Apollo could run faster still, and she soon saw that he was going to catch her. She set her teeth and tried to run still faster, but Apollo gained on her at every step. In despair she called to Mother Earth to save her from being taken. Immediately, a change came over Daphne. Her feet took root in the ground, her arms and fingers turned to branches and twigs, her dress became rough bark, and her lovely curling hair was changed to countless rustling leaves. When Apollo caught up to her she had become a beautiful laurel tree.

BAY

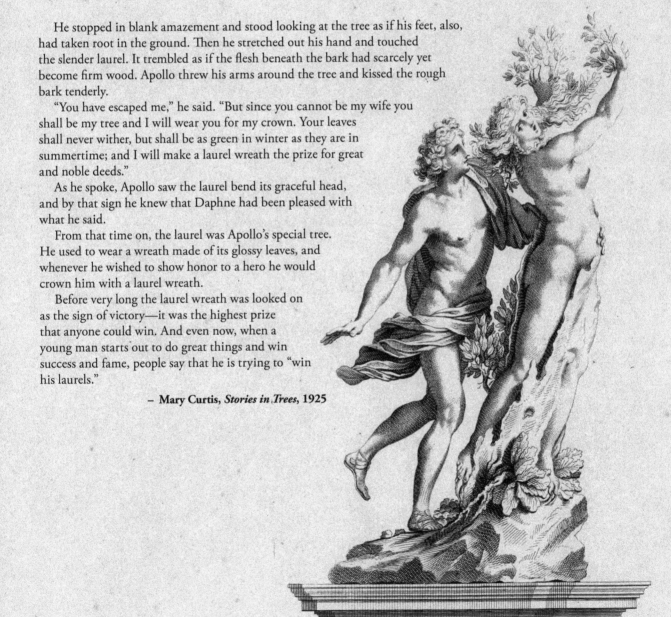

He stopped in blank amazement and stood looking at the tree as if his feet, also, had taken root in the ground. Then he stretched out his hand and touched the slender laurel. It trembled as if the flesh beneath the bark had scarcely yet become firm wood. Apollo threw his arms around the tree and kissed the rough bark tenderly.

"You have escaped me," he said. "But since you cannot be my wife you shall be my tree and I will wear you for my crown. Your leaves shall never wither, but shall be as green in winter as they are in summertime; and I will make a laurel wreath the prize for great and noble deeds."

As he spoke, Apollo saw the laurel bend its graceful head, and by that sign he knew that Daphne had been pleased with what he said.

From that time on, the laurel was Apollo's special tree. He used to wear a wreath made of its glossy leaves, and whenever he wished to show honor to a hero he would crown him with a laurel wreath.

Before very long the laurel wreath was looked on as the sign of victory—it was the highest prize that anyone could win. And even now, when a young man starts out to do great things and win success and fame, people say that he is trying to "win his laurels."

— **Mary Curtis**, *Stories in Trees*, 1925

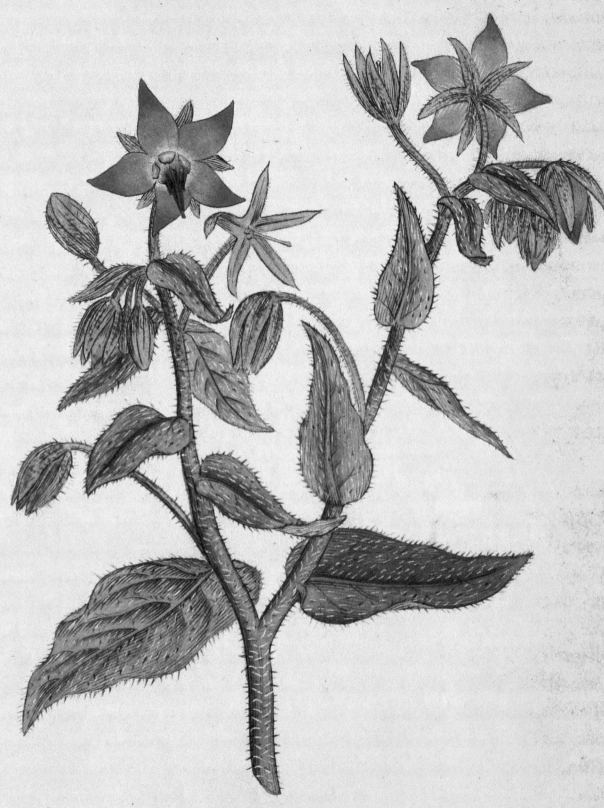

Borago officinalis

BORAGE

Other Names: **Starflower, Cool Tankard, Tailwort, Bee Bush, Bee Bread**
Latin Name: **Borago officinalis**
Symbolises: **Bluntness, courage**
Type: **Hardy annual**
Natural Habitat: **Aleppo, naturalised in Europe**
Growing Zone: **3–10**
Site: **Full sun or light shade**
Sow: **March to May**
Harvest: **June to September**
Usable Parts: **Leaves and flowers**
Companion Plants: **Balm and horehound**
Herbal Astrology: **Jupiter**

Originally hailing from the Mediterranean, borage makes an excellent border plant or gap filler for smaller gardens. Its beautiful blue, star-shaped flowers often adorn summer drinks and salads as a bright garnish. Much like its cheerful flowers, borage was used as a herbal remedy to lift one's spirit, earning it the nickname 'Herb of Gladness'.

The whole plant is rough with white, stiff, prickly hairs. The round stems, about 1 ½ feet high, are branched, hollow and succulent; the leaves alternate, large, wrinkled, deep green, oval and pointed, 3 inches long or more, and about 1 ½ inch broad, the lower ones stalked, with stiff, one celled hairs on the upper surfaces and on the veins below, the margins entire, but wavy. The flowers, which terminate the cells, are bright blue and star-shaped, distinguished from those of every plant in this order by their prominent black anthers, which form a cone in the centre and have been described as their beauty spot. The fruit consists of four brownish-black nutlets.

— **Maude Grieve, *A Modern Herbal*, 1931**

BORAGE

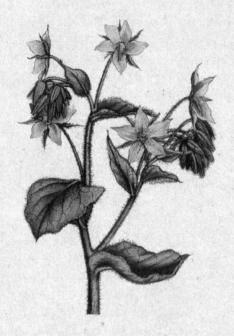

Borage and hellebore fill two scenes,
Sovereign plants to purge the veins
Of melancholy, and cheer the heart
Of those black fumes which make it smart;
To clear the brain of misty fogs,
Which dull our senses and Soul clogs;
The best medicine that e'er God made
For this malady, if well assay'd.

    – Robert Burton, *The Anatomy of Melancholy,* **1628**

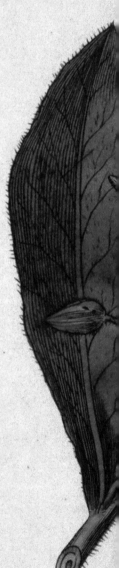

In the Garden

Coriander and Borage must be sowne in February or March, in a new Moone.

    – Richard Folkard, ***Plant Lore, Legends, and Lyrics,*** **1884**

Borage is an annual or biennial that once planted sows itself freely. Seed is planted in April and the seedlings thinned out to fifteen inches apart. It can also be increased by division in spring. In the herb garden Borage associates well with Balm and Horehound. The lush foliage of Balm in June contrasts well with the bristly leaves of Borage and the habit of growth of Horehound is a good foil for both.

    – Eleanour Sinclair Rohde, ***Herbs and Herb Gardening,*** **1936**

BORAGE

continued.

Ego Borago gaudia semper ago.

I Borage, bring always courage.

> **– John Gerard,** *The Herball; or, Generall Historie of Plantes,* **1597**

In the Kitchen

Those of our time do use the flowers in salads, to exhilarate and make the minde glad. There be also many things made of them, used for the comfort of the heart, to drive away sorrow & increase the joy of the minde.

> **– John Gerard,** *The Herball; or, Generall Historie of Plantes,* **1597**

The use of Borage in cups is very ancient, and old writers have ascribed to the flower many virtues. In Evelyn's Acetaria it is said "to revive the hypochondriac, and cheer the hard student." In Salmon's *Household Companion* (1710) Borage is mentioned as one of the four cordial flowers; "it comforts the heart, cheers melancholy, and revives the fainting spirits."

> **– John Bickerdyke,** *The Curiosities of Ale and Beer,* **1889**

In the early part of the nineteenth century, the young tops of Borage were still sometimes boiled as a pot-herb, and the young leaves were formerly considered good in salads.

The fresh herb has a cucumber-like fragrance. When steeped in water, it imparts a coolness to it and a faint cucumber flavour, and compounded with lemon and sugar in wine, and water, it makes a refreshing and restorative summer drink. It was formerly always an ingredient in cool tankards of wine and cider, and is still largely used in claret cup.

> **– Maude Grieve,** *A Modern Herbal,* **1931**

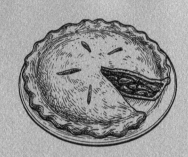

To Make a Tart of Borage Flowers, Marigolds or Cowslips

(From the Sixteenth Century)

This very interesting recipe comes from a *Proper Newe Booke of Cokerye* a black-letter book in the library of Corpus Christi College, Cambridge. This copy belonged to Archbishop Parker, and was edited by Miss Frere, and republished in 1913.

1. Take borage flowers and parboil them tender.

2. Then strain them and

3. Mix them with the yolks of 3—4 eggs and sweet curds.

4. Or else take 3—4 apples and parboil them, and strain them and mix them with sweet butter and the yolks of eggs and a little mace and so bake it.

[N.B.— In those days it would be baked in a raised pastry coffin. To-day it would be baked in a fireproof glass piedish.—ED.]

– **Florence White,** *Good Things in England,* **1932**

BORAGE

continued.

ANCIENT KNOWLEDGE, VIRTUES, AND LORE

Medicinal Properties and Remedies

The belief that the herb had power to dispel melancholy was universal. In Welsh its name 'Llawenlys' signifies 'Herb of Gladness' and Gerard says: 'Those of our time do use the flowers in salads to exhilarate and make the mind glad.' Bacon assures us that 'the leaf of the borage hath an excellent spirit to repress the fuliginous vapour of dusky melancholy.'

— **Sabine Baring-Gould**, *An Old English Home and Its Dependencies*, **1898**

Borage Remedy for Hydration & Fever

A Remedie to take away the drought in an ague

TAKE Sorell and Borrage, of each of them a like quantitie, and a certaine quantitie of Strawberrie leaves, & Violet leaves, boyle them altogether in a pottle of very faire running water, until it be consumed from a pottle to a quarte, then take the Hearbes and straine them, and then take halfe a pound of good Almondes, and blanche them, & beate and straine them with the saide water, and put Sugar therein, and drinke it warme, do this for the space of five or sixe daies, and it will help him.

— **A. T.**, *A Rich Storehouse or Treasurie for the Diseased*, **1616**

Folk Beliefs

But, to quote another kind of sympathy between human beings and certain plants, the Cingalese have a notion that the cocoa-nut plant withers away when beyond the reach of a human voice, and that the vervain and borage will only thrive near man's dwellings.

— **Thomas Firminger Thistelton-Dyer**, *The Folk-lore of Plants*, **1889**

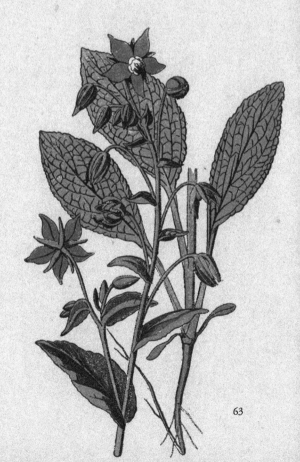

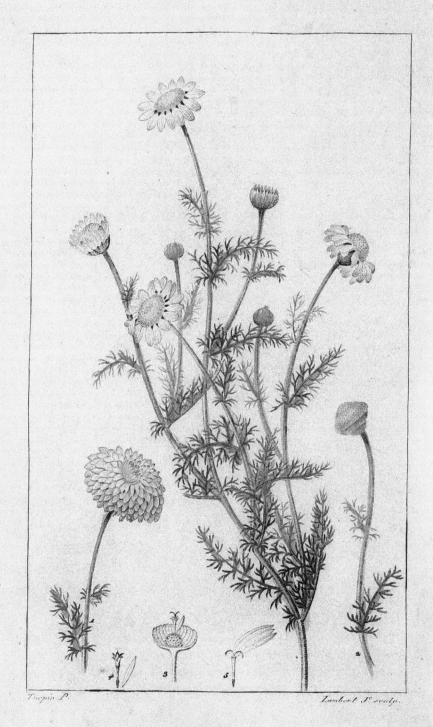

Turpin P.   Lambert F. sculp.

CAMOMILLE.

a.l.l.

CHAMOMILE

Other Names: Common Chamomile, Camomile
Latin Name: Chamaemelum nobile, Anthemis nobilis
Symbolises: Energy in adversity
Type: Hardy perennial
Natural Habitat: Europe, including Great Britain
Growing Zone: 3–9
Site: Blooms best in full sun, but will grow in partial shade
Sow: March to April in well-drained soil
Harvest: August to October in full bloom
Usable Parts: Flower
Companion Plants: Basil or brassicas
Herbal Astrology: The Sun

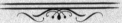

The calming properties of this flower have been used in folk medicine for centuries, with chamomile tea often a favourite choice for those looking to improve their sleep. One of the most ancient medicinal herbs known, the delicate, daisy-like flowers have been employed for treating ailments from the common cold to snake bites. An easy grower with charming flora, it was once regarded as a blessing from the gods due to its abundant virtues.

Chamomile is one of the oldest favourites amongst garden herbs and its reputation as a medicinal plant shows little signs of abatement. The Egyptians reverenced it for its virtues and from their belief in its power to cure ague, dedicated it to their gods. No plant was better known to the country folk of old, it having been grown for centuries in English gardens for its use as a common domestic medicine.

– Maude Grieve, *A Modern Herbal*, 1931

CHAMOMILE

continued.

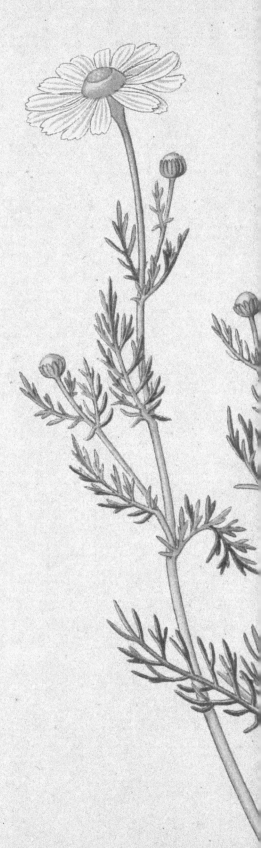

Whilst some still busied are in decking of the bride,
Some others were again as seriously imploy'd
In strewing of those hearbs at bridalls us'd that be
Which everywhere they throwe with bountious hands and free
The healthfull balme and mint, from their full laps doe fly
The sent-full camomill, the verdurous Costmary.

> – **Michael Drayton,** *The Poly-Olbion,* 1612

Like a chamomile bed –
The more it is trodden
The more it will spread

> – **Maude Grieve,** *A Modern Herbal,* 1931

…The fragrant chamomile, that spreads
  Its leaflets fresh and green,
And richly broiders every niche
  The velvet turf between…

> – **Lydia Huntley Sigourney, 'Planting Flowers on the**
> **Grave of Parents',** 1841

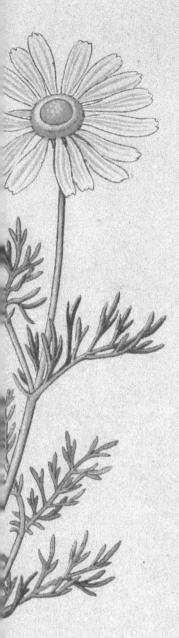

CHAMOMILE continued.

In the Garden

Each old plant in March is divided into ten or twelve portions: these are planted in rows 2 1/2 feet apart, with a distance of 18 inches between the plants in the row. The flowers are picked in September, rapidly dried, and laid on canvas trays in a heated drying-closet.

— **David Ellis,** *Medicinal Herbs and Poisonous Plants,* **1918**

In the Kitchen

The flowers, which are the parts generally used, are in high repute, both in the popular and scientific materia medica, and give out their properties by infusion in either water or alcohol. The flowers are also used in the manufacture of bitter beer, and along with wormwood are used to a certain extent as a substitute for hops. It is considered a safe bitter and tonic, though strong infusions, when taken warm, act sometimes as an emetic.

— **Jules Arthur Harder,** *The Physiology of Taste,* **1885**

ANCIENT KNOWLEDGE, VIRTUES, AND LORE

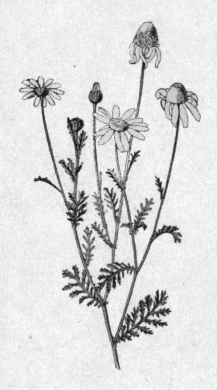

Medicinal Properties and Remedies

Being a tonic, it strengthens the stomach when drunk in the morning. It is externally discutient; emollient when used for callouses, shrunken sinews, gout, enlarged joints, and white swellings. The warm tea promotes the operation of emetics; intermittents, dyspepsia, hysteria, flatulent colic; as fomentations in gripings; and to ripen suppurating tumours.

– **Nicholas Culpeper & William Joseph Simmonite,** *Herbal Remedies of Culpeper and Simmonite,* **1957**

Chamomile Tea should in all cases be prepared in a covered vessel, in order to prevent the escape of steam, as the medicinal value of the flowers is to a considerable extent impaired by any evaporation, and the infusion should be allowed to stand on the flowers for 10 minutes at least before straining off.

Combined with ginger and alkalies, the cold infusion (made with ½ oz of flowers to 1 pint of water) proves an excellent stomachic in cases of ordinary indigestion, such as flatulent colic, heartburn, loss of appetite, sluggish state of the intestinal canal, and also in gout and periodic headache, and is an appetizing tonic, especially for aged persons, taken an hour or more before a principal meal. A strong, warm infusion is a useful emetic. A concentrated infusion made eight times as strong as the ordinary infusion, is made from the powdered flowers with oil of chamomile and alcohol given as a stomachic in doses of ½ to 2 drachms, three times daily.

Apart from their use internally, Chamomile flowers are also extensively used by themselves, or combined with an equal quantity of crushed poppy-heads, as a poultice and fomentation for external swelling, inflammatory pain or congested neuralgia, and will relieve where other remedies have failed, proving invaluable for reducing swellings of the face caused through abscesses. Bags may be stuffed with flowers and steeped well in boiling water before being applied as a fomentation. The antiseptic powers of Chamomile are stated to be 120 times stronger than sea-water.

– **Maude Grieve,** *A Modern Herbal,* **1931**

[In spring] medical men pound the leaves, and make them up into lozenges, the same being done with the flowers also, and the root. All the parts of this plant are administered together, in doses of one drachma, for the stings of serpents of all kinds.

– Elder Pliny, *The Natural History of Pliny*, c. 77 AD

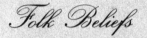

Folk Beliefs

According to Galen, the Egyptians held the Chamomile (Anthemis nobilis) in such reverence, that they consecrated it to their deities: they had great faith in the plant as a remedy for agues. Gerarde tells us that Chamomile is a special help against wearisomeness, and that it derives its name from the Greek Chamaimelon, Earth-Apple, because the flowers have the smell of an Apple.—In Germany, Chamomile-flowers are called Heermännchen, and they are traditionally supposed to have once been soldiers, who for their sins died accursed.—The Romans supposed the Anthemis to be possessed of properties to cure the bites of serpents.

– Richard Folkard, *Plant Lore, Legends, and Lyrics*, 1884

The following anecdote of Mrs. Elliott has been mentioned. An officer of- the royal army, noted for his cruelty and relentless persecution of those opposed to his political views, was one day walking with her in a garden where was a great variety of flowers. " What is this, madam?" he asked, pointing to the chamomile.

"The rebel flower," she replied. " And why is it called the rebel flower?" asked the 'officer. "Because," answered Mrs. Elliott, "it always flourishes most when trampled upon."

– Elizabeth F. Ellet, *The Women of the American Revolution*, 1849

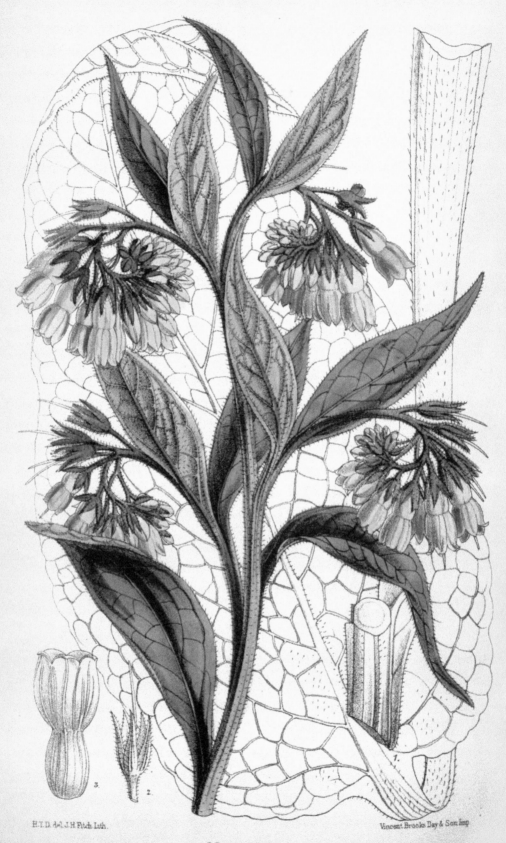

H.T.D. del. J.H. Fitch Lith.

Vincent Brooks Day & Son Imp

L. Reeve & C⁰ London.

COMFREY

Other Names: Healing Herb, Bone-knit, Boneset, Bruisewort, Knit Bone
Latin Name: Symphytum officinale
Symbolises: Prosperity
Type: Perennial
Natural Habitat: Europe
Growing Zone: 4–8
Site: Plant in the ground in full sun
Sow: March to June
Harvest: Best to harvest in its second season
Cut in autumn, no later than September
Usable Parts: Young leaves and buds
Companion Plants: Marigolds
Herbal Astrology: Saturn

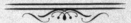

Grown prolifically in kitchen gardens as a fertiliser full of essential nutrients, comfrey's clusters of purple bell flowers are a decorative and practical addition to any plot. The charming blooms resemble the poisonous foxglove and grow just as abundantly when planted. While recent studies warn against eating the plant due to its toxic properties, it can also effectively remedy swelling or bruising when applied externally as an ointment. If not grown for healing, use it in your garden as a fertiliser in your compost or liquid feed.

One of the most attractive of physic herbs and one of the earliest in bloom. It varies in height from eighteen inches in poor soil to nearly three feet in rich, moist soil and in the south and sheltered parts its pretty, bugle-like flowers are produced in April. The type has cream-coloured flowers but there is a variety with purplish flowers. The dwarf form is frequently in flower as early as February.

– **Eleanour Sinclair Rohde,** *Herbs and Herb Gardening,* **1936**

This handsome plant, with its yellow, pink or purple, drooping flowers, and large, elliptical, hairy, pointed leaves, is common in watery places and on the banks of rivers. Another striking feature are the wings which line the upper part of the stem.

– **David Ellis,** *Medicinal Herbs and Poisonous Plants,* **1918**

This wort strengthens the man.

– **Charles J. MacAlister,** *Comfrey – An Ancient Medicinal Remedy,* **1936**

COMFREY

continued.

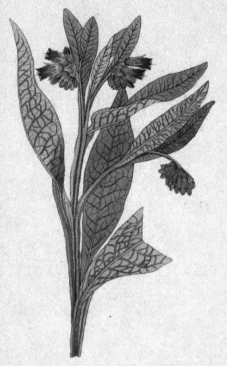

In the Garden

In the herb garden Comfrey associates well with Marigolds, for Comfrey is in full beauty early in the year and in summer and autumn the foliage helps to support the Marigold stalks. Comfrey is a perennial and is easily increased by root division in autumn. It flourishes in any soil.

— **Eleanour Sinclair Rohde,** *Herbs and Herb Gardening,* **1936**

The cultivation of the herb is a very easy matter, and in many cases the difficulty is to prevent it from spreading over the whole garden, after it has once got a good start; the smallest bit of root left in the ground will grow, and raise a fresh colony. The leaves are collected in May, and the roots in July.

— **David Ellis,** *Medicinal Herbs and Poisonous Plants,* **1918**

In the Kitchen

In cookery, the leaves gathered young may be used as a substitute for spinach; the young shoots have been eaten after blanching by forcing them to grow through heaps of earth.

— **Maude Grieve,** *A Modern Herbal,* **1931**

ANCIENT KNOWLEDGE, VIRTUES, AND LORE

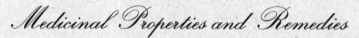

Medicinal Properties and Remedies

The names by which it was popularly known. For instance Knitbacke (Gerrard 1597), Comfort Knitbene (Scotland). In Aberdeen it was called Comfer Knitbeen, and a preparation made by boiling the root in oil or lard was extolled by old women for hardening and strengthening fractures. This property also accounted for its being called Bone-set or Knit Bone in Lancashire. It appears to have been used both internally and externally in fractures in all districts.

— **Charles J. MacAlister,** *Comfrey – An Ancient Medicinal Remedy,* **1936**

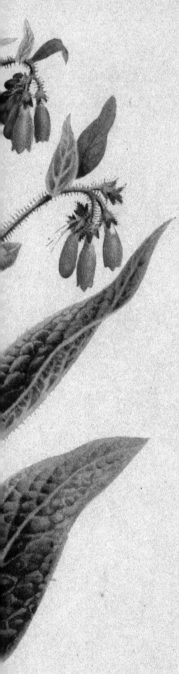

COMFREY

continued.

Take of Comfrey Root 6 ounces; Plantain leaves, 3 ounces. Bruise together in a marble mortar to express the juice; strain the liquid and add an equal quantity of sugar (…) to be taken in doses of 2 tablespoonfuls; this is also good for coughs by adding an ounce or two of liquorice-root. The beaten root is laid on leather and applied to parts affected with gout, rheumatism, and other pains in the joints.

– **Nicholas Culpeper & William Joseph Simmonite,** *Herbal Remedies of Culpeper and Simmonite,* **1957**

It has long been employed domestically in lung troubles and also for quinsy and whooping-cough. The root is more effectual than the leaves and is the part usually used in cases of coughs (…) A modern medicinal tincture, employed by homoeopaths, is made from the root with spirits of wine, 10 drops in a tablespoon of water being administered several times a day.

– **Maude Grieve,** *A Modern Herbal,* **1931**

Folk Beliefs

When visiting a farm at Tarvin in Cheshire many years ago, I was interested to find that its owner always kept a bed of comfrey in order that he might provide villagers with it when occasions arose. Dr. Walter Moore, of Bourton-on-the-Water, has recently informed me that, within his recollection, plots of it were grown as a food for cattle, on account of its reputation for producing milk, rich broth in quality and quantity. Another interesting Gloucestershire reference is contained in a letter published by Mr. Edwin Green of Cheltenham (Daily Mail, March 27, 1912) in which he wrote that (…) He knew a gentleman near Cheltenham who had a field of 4 acres in which nothing but his plant was grown. He gave it not only to his horses but was never without a dish of it, when in season, instead of spinach.

(…)

I myself have heard Comfrey spoken of as an "old woman's remedy", and I admit it in the sense that it probably dates from the time when woman was the priestess of Medicine. (…) "She was the Witch or Wise Woman of those days— and it is within the realms of possibility that comfrey was among the "simples" employed by her, and may truly be called an old or ancient "woman's remedy."

– **Charles J. MacAlister,** *Comfrey – An Ancient Medicinal Remedy,* **1936**

Tab. 6

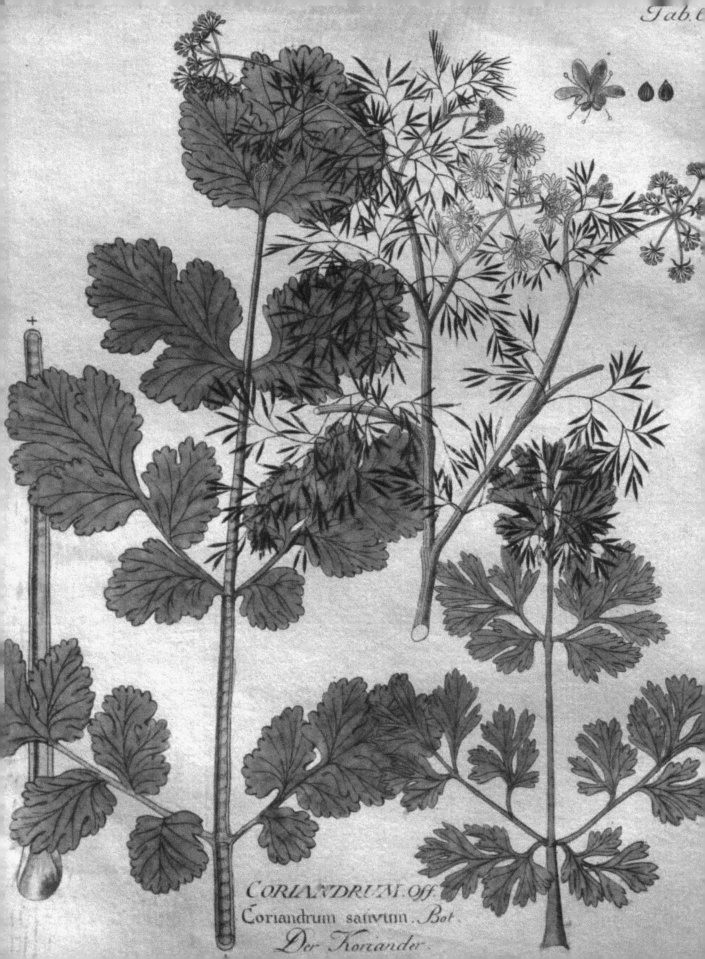

CORIANDRUM. Off.
Coriandrum sativum. Bot.
Der Koriander.

CORIANDER

Other Names: Cilantro
Latin Name: Coriandrum sativum
Symbolises: Hidden worth
Type: Hardy annual
Natural Habitat: Eastern Mediterranean and southern Europe
Growing Zone: 2–11
Site: Outdoor in lightly shaded spot
Sow: March to October
Harvest: From June onwards. Regular picking encourages
new leaves
Usable Parts: Leaves, stem, and seeds
Companion Plants: Basil, chervil, dill, parsley, spinach, and tomatoes
Herbal Astrology: Mars

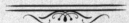

Whether you love or hate it, the fragrant coriander is a well-used ingredient in the modern kitchen, with its punchy flavour embellishing dishes from all over the world. More recently, it has been scientifically proven that the taste and smell of coriander can differ depending on your genetic makeup, with some brandishing it soap-like on the palette.

A hardy annual, growing about 2 feet high, and bearing white flowers in June or later, according to the time of sowing.

– David Ellis, *Medicinal Herbs and Poisonous Plants,* 1918

A native of Southern Europe. It is taller growing than either Caraway or Anise, indeed, Gerard describes it as "a very striking herb". It attains about three feet and flowers in July. Seed is sown either in spring or autumn. The tiny, round seeds have a very disagreeable scent, when fresh, but the longer they are kept the more aromatic they become.

– Eleanour Sinclair Rohde, *Herbs and Herb Gardening,* 1936

CORIANDER

continued.

And Coriander last to these succeeds
That hangs on slightest threads her trembling seeds.

> – **William Cowper, 'The Salad. By Virgil', 1799**

In the Garden

Sow in mild, dry weather in April, in shallow drills, about 1/2 inch deep and 8 or 9 inches apart, and cover it evenly with the soil. The seeds are slow in germinating. The seeds may also be sown in March, in heat, for planting out in May.

As the seeds ripen, about August, the disagreeable odour gives place to a pleasant aroma, and the plant is then cut down with sickles and when dry the fruit is threshed out.

> – **Maude Grieve,** *A Modern Herbal,* **1931**

In the Kitchen

The seeds have been used as a condiment from very ancient times. Manna was compared to Coriander seed—"And the house of Israel called the name thereof Manna, and it was like Coriander seed, white, and the taste of it was like wafers made with honey." This is the only mention of Coriander in the Bible. The Israelites must have been very familiar with Coriander, for the best Coriander, according to Pliny, came from Egypt. It was cultivated in this country in very early times and is mentioned in Jon Gardener's Feate of Gardening, 1440. Formerly it was grown commercially in this country, but our main supplies now come from Holland and Russia. Coriander is still a favourite condiment in the East and is an ingredient in curry powder.

> – **Eleanour Sinclair Rohde,** *Herbs and Herb Gardening,* **1936**

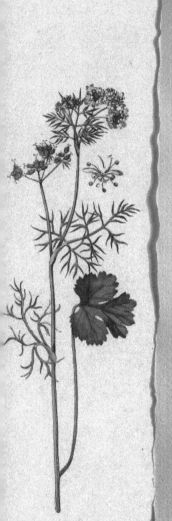

Juniper Cordial

Ingredients:

15g dried Juniper Berries
225ml Water
One bunch of Coriander
225ml Sugar Syrup

Method:

1. Crush the juniper berries in a large (sterilised) jar, and add the water.

2. Add the coriander and sugar syrup and shake well.

3. Allow the mixture to stand for two weeks then carefully strain the liquid through a clean muslin cloth.

4. Pour into sterilised bottles to store.

– Two Magpies Publishing, *A-Z of Homemade Syrups and Cordials,* **2014**

CORIANDER

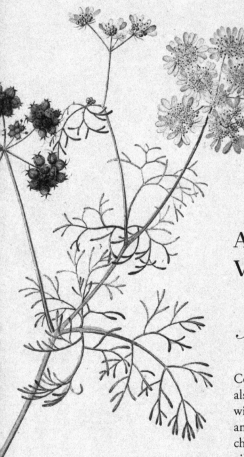

ANCIENT KNOWLEDGE, VIRTUES, AND LORE

Medicinal Properties and Remedies

While green, it is possessed of very cooling and refreshing properties. Combined with honey or raisins, it is an excellent remedy for spreading ulcers, as also for diseases of the testes, burns, carbuncles, and maladies of the ears. Applied with woman's milk, it is good for defluxions of the eyes; and for fluxes of the belly and intestines, the seed is taken with water in drink; it is also taken in drink for cholera, with rue. Coriander seed, used as a potion with pomegranate juice and oil, expels worms in the intestines.

– Elder Pliny, *The Natural History of Pliny,* **c. 77 AD**

A Remedy for one who vomiteth too much – Take Coriander seeds fine beaten in powder, and drink it with Mint water.

– Hugh Plat, *Delights for Ladies to Adorn their Persons, Tables, Closets, and Distillatories,* **1644**

The leaves and seeds being green, are cold and dry, and hurtful to the body, if taken inwardly; but the seeds being steeped in Vinegar, and dryed, are moderately hot and dry, and then they are good for the Stomach, and helps digestion: the Comfits of the prepared seeds repress Vapours that ascend to the head, help digestion, and stay vomiting. The seeds taken in Wine, kills Worms, and stops Fluxes, helps the Winde Chollick, and stopping of urine. The powder of the seed drunk in sweet Wine, provokes lust, the green herb boiled with Barley meal, helps Inflammations.

– Robert Turner, *Botanologia the British Physician: Or, The Vertues of English Plants,* **1664**

CORIANDER

continued.

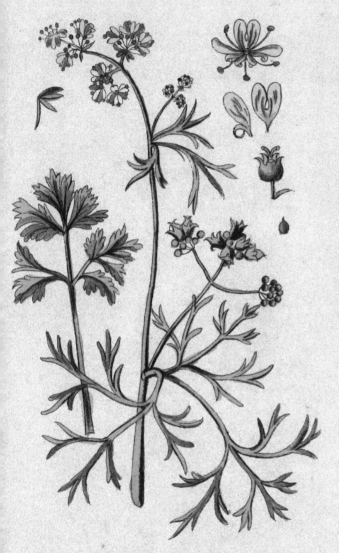

Folk Beliefs

Coriander was originally introduced from the East, being one of the herbs brought to Britain by the Romans. As an aromatic stimulant and spice, it has been cultivated and used from very ancient times. It was employed by Hippocrates and other Greek physicians.

The name Coriandrum, used by Pliny, is derived from *koros*, (a bug), in reference to the foetid smell of the leaves.

Pliny tells us that 'the best (coriander) came from Egypt,' and thence no doubt the Israelites grained their knowledge of its properties.

The Africans are said to have called this herb by a similar name (goid), which Gesenius derives from a verd (gadad), signifying 'to cut', in an allusion to the furrowed appearance of the fruit.

A power of conferring immortality is thought by the Chinese to be a property of the seeds.

– Maude Grieve, *A Modern Herbal,* 1931

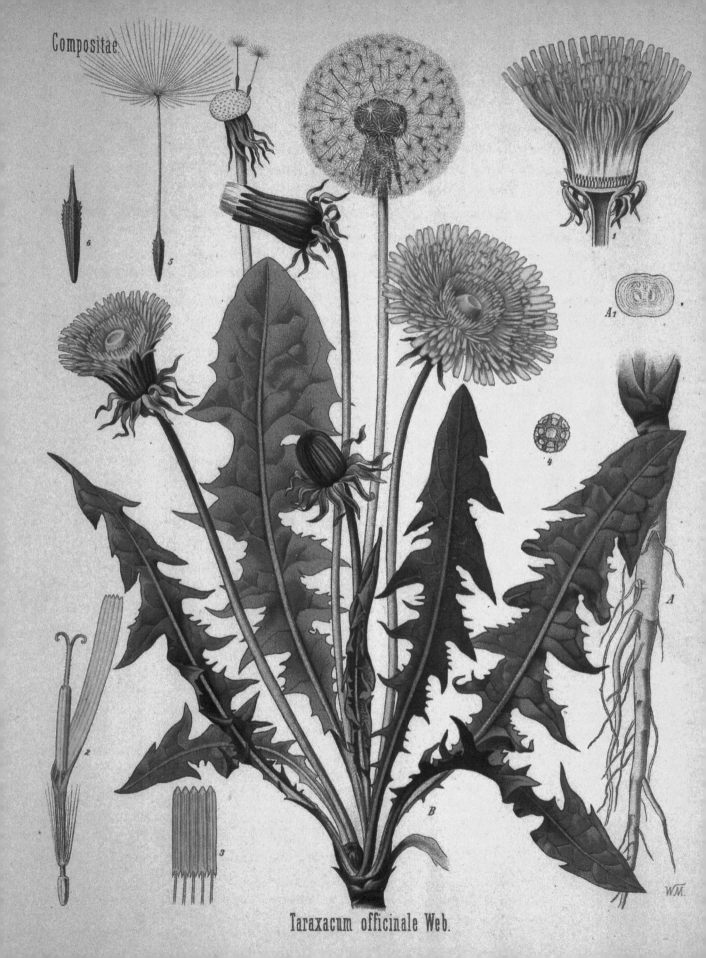

Compositae.

Taraxacum officinale Web.

DANDELION

Other Names: Swine Snout, Puff Ball, Lion's Tooth,
White Wild Endive, Priest's Crown
Latin Name: Leontodon taraxacum
Symbolises: Rustic article
Type: Perennial
Natural Habitat: All temperate regions
Growing Zone: 3–9
Site: Outside in well-drained soil
Sow: February to March
Harvest: March to October
Usable Parts: Leaves, stem, flower, and root
Companion Plants: Beans, clover, and tomatoes
Herbal Astrology: Jupiter

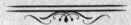

*Commonly found sprinkled across fields, gardens, and verges, the cheerful
dandelion is often regarded as a weed despite its reputation as a traditional medicine.
Humans have eaten its yellow flowers for much of recorded history, while the roots
can be dried and made into an excellent substitute for coffee. After transforming
from bright yellow flowers to fluffy seed heads, the delicate spheres were often used as
nature's clock, and it is said that when blown, one could tell the time.*

It is [the] somewhat fanciful resemblance to the canine teeth of a lion that (it is
generally assumed) gives the plant its most familiar name of Dandelion, which is
a corruption of the French Dent de Lion, an equivalent of this name being found
not only in its former specific Latin name Dens leonis and in the Greek name
for the genus to which Linnaeus assigned it, Leontodon, but also in nearly all the
languages of Europe.

– Maude Grieve, *A Modern Herbal*, 1931

DANDELION

continued.

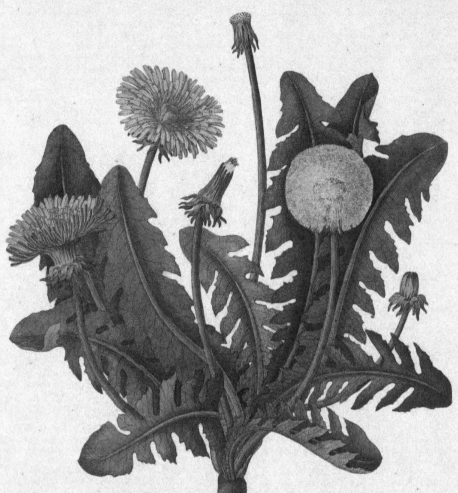

Dear common flower, that grow'st beside the way,
Fringing the dusty road with harmless gold,
   First pledge of blithesome May,
Which children pluck, and, full of pride, uphold,
  High-hearted buccaneers, o'erjoyed that they
An Eldorado in the grass have found,
   Which not the rich earth's ample round
May match in wealth,—thou art more dear to me
Than all the prouder summer-blooms may be.

    – James Russell Lowell, 'To the Dandelion', 1865

Dandelion, with globe and down,
The schoolboy's clock in every town,
Which the truant puffs amain,
To conjure lost hours back again.

    – William Howitt, *The Book*
    of Herbs, **1903**

The dandelions and buttercups
Gild all the lawn; the drowsy bee
Stumbles among the clover-tops,
And summer sweetens all but me.

    – John Burroughs, *Pepacton,* **1871**

DANDELION

continued.

In the Garden

When cultivated the seeds should be sown in May or June, in drills half an inch deep and twelve inches apart. The plants will be ready for use the following spring. It is also extensively grown for its roots. For this purpose it is sown in September and cultivated well during the fall, and in the following season the roots will be fit to dig up in October. The roots, after being dried, constitute an article of commercial importance, being extensively employed as a substitute for, or mixed with coffee.

– Jules Arthur Harder, *The Physiology of Taste,* **1885**

In the Kitchen

The young leaves should be picked before the plant flowers, and treated as. It mixes well with other saladings. Also it may be boiled in water, seasoned with butter, and served as a vegetable. Those plants which have been covered with earth by moles are nicely blanched, and make a more appetising salad. It is obtainable during the winter months.

– L. C. R. Cameron, *The Wild Foods of Great Britain,* **1917**

Dandelion Coffee

In the spring-time, when the dandelion has flowered and is at its best, the roots are dug up, washed, and dried in the sun. They are then cut into pieces, these pieces placed in a tin and roasted over the hot embers of a fire, pounded on a heavy stone, rubbed carefully through a sieve, and put in a tin and stored for the winter.

– Gipsy Petulengro, *A Romany Life,* **1935**

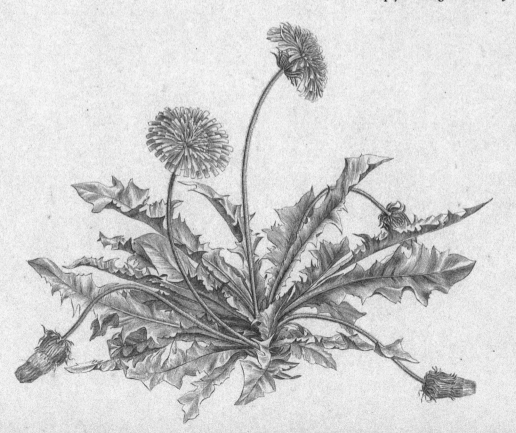

Dandelion Cordial

Ingredients

100g (or slightly more) Dandelion Heads
650ml Water
450g Sugar
2 Oranges
2 Lemons
A handful of Raisins

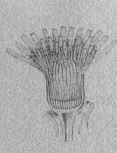

Method

1. Place the dandelions in a large bowl and cover with the boiling water.

2. Allow this mixture to stand for three days, then filter through a clean muslin cloth.

3. Place the liquid in a sterilised bottle with the dissolved sugar, and strained juice of the lemons and oranges.

4. Allow this mixture to stand for at least three days.

5. Decant into smaller bottles to store and (if you like), place two raisins in each bottle before sealing. This will impart a rounder, sweeter flavour.

– **Two Magpies Publishing,** *A-Z of Homemade Syrups and Cordials,* **2014**

DANDELION
 continued.

Simple and fresh and fair from winter's close emerging,
As if no artifice of fashion, business, politics, had ever been,
Forth from its sunny nook of shelter'd grass - innocent, golden,
  calm as the dawn,
The spring's first dandelion shows its trustful face.

– Walt Whitman, 'The First Dandelion', 1888

ANCIENT KNOWLEDGE, VIRTUES, AND LORE

Medicinal Properties and Remedies

Dandelion (…) was used as an effective laxative and diuretic, and as a treatment for bile or liver problems.

– David Ellis, *Medicinal Herbs and Poisonous Plants*, 1918

It is of an opening and cleansing quality, and therefore very effectual for the obstructions of the liver, gall and spleen, and the diseases that arise from them, as the jaundice and hypocondriac; it opens the passages of the urine both in young and old; powerfully cleanses imposthumes and inward ulcers in the urinary passage, and by its drying and temperate quality doth afterwards heal them; for which purpose the decoction of the roots or leaves in white wine, or the leaves chopped as pot-herbs, with a few Alisanders, and boiled in their broth, are very effectual. And whoever is drawing towards a consumption or an evil disposition of the whole body, called Cachexia, by the use hereof for some time together, shall find a wonderful help. It helps also to procure rest and sleep to bodies distempered by the heat of ague fits, or otherwise: The distilled water is effectual to drink in pestilential fevers, and to wash the sores.

– Nicholas Culpeper, *Complete Herbal*, 1824

DANDELION COFFEE. Is prepared from selected English roots properly ground and correctly roasted. Its value in the case of Kidney and Liver troubles as well as to the digestion, is too well known to need emphasis.

– King Press, *The Famous Book of Herbs*, 2013

85

Herbal Magic

To dream you are gathering dandelions, and the flowers seem fresh, the dream shows you will have a letter from someone of whom you are thinking. But a large bed of dandelions is a warning of a new enemy.

— **Diana Hawthorne,** *Laurie's Complete Fortune Teller,* **1946**

For the heartbeat there's nothing so good as dandelion. There was a woman I knew used to boil it down, and she'd throw out what was left on the grass. And there was a fleet of turkeys about the house and they used to be picking it up. And at Christmas they killed one of them, and when it was cut open they found a new heart growing in it with the dint of the dandelion.

— **Augusta Gregory,** *Visions and Beliefs in the West of Ireland,* **1920**

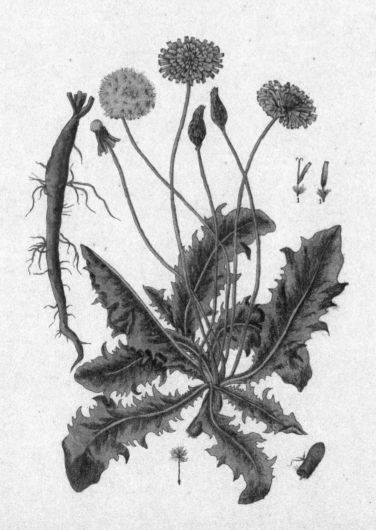

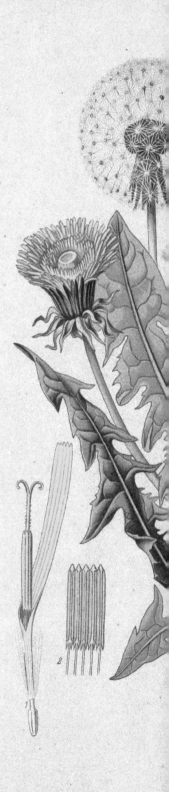

DANDELION continued.

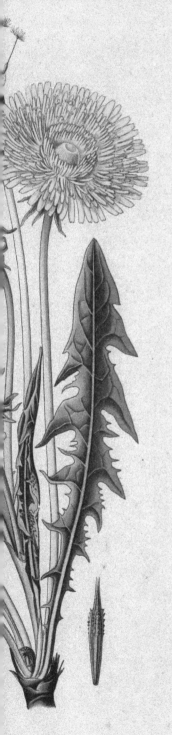

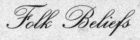

Dandelions close their blossoms before a storm. When the down of the dandelion contracts, it is a sign of rain.

— **David Bowen**, *Folklore Guide to the Weather,* **1953**

Certainly in appearance of the Dandelion-flower is very suggestive of the ancient representations of the sun. In German Switzerland, the children form chains of the stalks of Dandelions, and holding the garland in their hands, they dance round and round in a circle. The Dandelion is called the rustic oracle: its flowers always open about five a.m. and shut at eight p.m., serving the shepherd for a clock —

"Leontodons unfold
On the swart turf their ray-encircled gold,
With Sol's expanding beam the flowers unclose,
And rising Hesper lights them to repose." — *Darwin.*

As the flower is the shepherd's clock, so are the feathery seed-tufts his barometer, predicting calm or storm. These downy seed-balls, which children blow off to find out the hour of the day, serve for other oracular purposes. Are you separated from the object of your love? – carefully pluck one of the feathery heads, charge each of the little feathers composing it with a tender thought; turn towards the spot where the loved one dwells; blow, and the seed ball will convey your message faithfully. Do you wish to know if that dear one is thinking of you, blow again; and if there be left upon the stalk a single aigrette, it is proof you are not forgotten. Similarly the Dandelion is consulted as to whether the lover lives east, west, north or south, and whether he is coming or not.

"Will he come? I pluck the flower leaves off,
    And each, cry, yes – no – yes;
I blow the down from the dry Hawkweed,
    Once, twice – hah! It flies amiss!" – *Scott.*

— **Richard Folkard**, *Plant Lore, Legends, and Lyrics,* **1884**

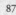

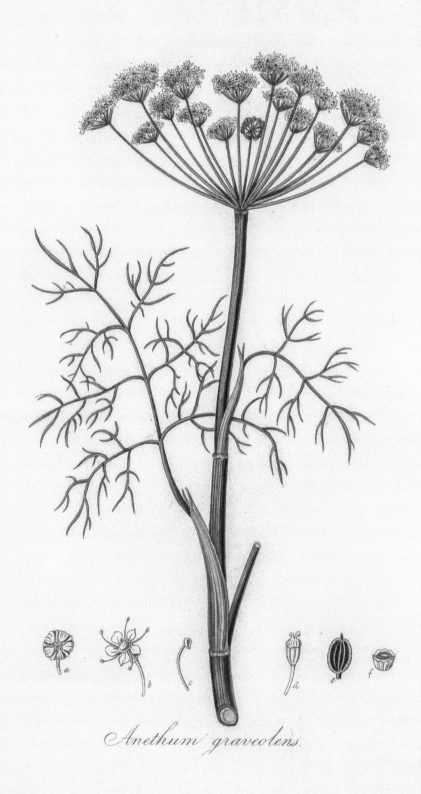

Anethum graveolens.

DILL

Other Names: Dill Weed, Dillweed, Suva Bhaji
Latin Name: Peucedanum graveolens
Symbolises: Good fortune
Type: Tender Annual
Natural Habitat: Southern Russia and countries bordering the Mediterranean
Growing Zone: 2–11
Site: Full sun
Sow: February to May, or September
Harvest: Anytime, just before it starts to flower
Usable Parts: Leaves and stem
Companion Plants: Chives, lemon balm, lemon thyme, and lovage
Herbal Astrology: Mercury

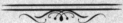

Another delicate culinary herb, dill features in many Scandinavian recipes to flavour things such as salmon and potato dishes. While packing a nutritional punch, its anti-inflammatory qualities have been praised since the time of Gerrard and Culpeper. Although it is primarily used in the kitchen today, its past is steeped in magical folklore, regularly applied as a defence against dark magic and evil forces.

The common Dill grows up with seldom more than one stalk, neither so high, nor so great usually as Fennel, being round and fewer joints thereon, whose leaves are sadder, and somewhat long, and so like Fennel that it deceives many, but harder in handling, and somewhat thicker, and of a strong unpleasant scent: The tops of the stalks have four branches and smaller umbels of yellow flowers, which turn into small seed, somewhat flatter and thinner than Fennel seed.

– Nicholas Culpeper, *Complete Herbal*, 1824

DILL

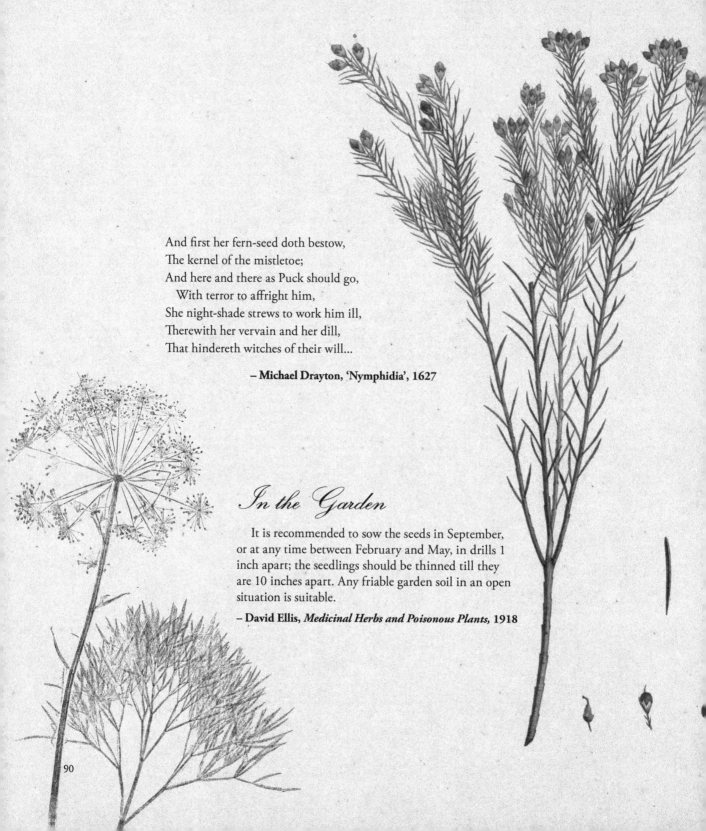

And first her fern-seed doth bestow,
The kernel of the mistletoe;
And here and there as Puck should go,
    With terror to affright him,
She night-shade strews to work him ill,
Therewith her vervain and her dill,
That hindereth witches of their will...

– Michael Drayton, 'Nymphidia', 1627

In the Garden

It is recommended to sow the seeds in September,
or at any time between February and May, in drills 1
inch apart; the seedlings should be thinned till they
are 10 inches apart. Any friable garden soil in an open
situation is suitable.

– David Ellis, *Medicinal Herbs and Poisonous Plants,* **1918**

In the Kitchen

Pickled Gherkins

Ingredients:

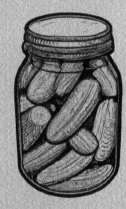

1 kg gherkins (small cucumbers)
300g salt
700ml white vinegar
700ml water
2 cloves of garlic
2 sprigs of dill
2 tbsps coriander seeds

Method:

1. Ensure the gherkins are clean and presentable, then gently prick them with a fork.

2. Place the gherkins, along with the salt into a large, ceramic or glass bowl and combine thoroughly.

3. Leave this mixture to infuse for at least four hours. This process will result in a 'crisper' end pickle, as the salt dehydrates them.

4. Once the gherkins have infused with the salt, wash them thoroughly in cold water.

5. Take a large, heavy-bottomed sauce pan and add the vinegar, water, chopped garlic, dill and coriander.

6. Cook very briefly on a low heat - to allow the flavours to combine.

7. Add the gherkins to the vinegar solution, and place in sterilise glass jars. Cover with a wax paper disc and seal.

– **Two Magpies Publishing,** *The A-Z of Homemade Chutneys, Pickles, and Relishes,* **2014**

DILL

continued.

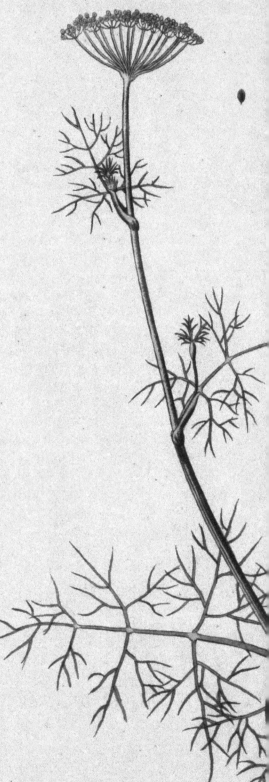

ANCIENT KNOWLEDGE, VIRTUES, AND LORE

Medicinal Properties and Remedies

Dill acts also as a carminative, allays gripings of the stomach, and arrests looseness of the bowels. The roots of this plant are applied topically in water, or else in wine, for defluxions of the eyes. The seed of it, if smelt at while boiling, will arrest hiccup; and, taken in water, it dispels indigestion. The ashes of it are a remedy for swellings of the uvula; but the plant itself weakens the eyesight and the generative powers.

– **Elder Pliny,** *The Natural History of Pliny,* c. 77 AD

The seed is of more use than the leaves, and more effectual to digest raw and vicious humours, and is used in medicines that serve to expel wind, and the pains proceeding therefrom. The seed, being roasted or fried, and used in oils or plasters, dissolve the imposthumes in the fundament; and dries up all moist ulcers, especially in the fundament; an oil made of Dill is effectual to warm or dissolve humours and imposthumes, and the pains, and to procure rest. The decoction of Dill, be it herb or seed (only if you boil the seed you must bruise it) in white wine, being drank, it is a gallant expeller of wind, and provoker of the terms.

– **Nicholas Culpeper,** *Complete Herbal,* 1824

Oil of dill is used in mixtures, or administered in doses of 5 drops on sugar, but its most common use is in the preparation of Dill water, which is a common domestic remedy for the flatulence of infants.

– **Maude Grieve,** *A Modern Herbal,* 1931

DILL

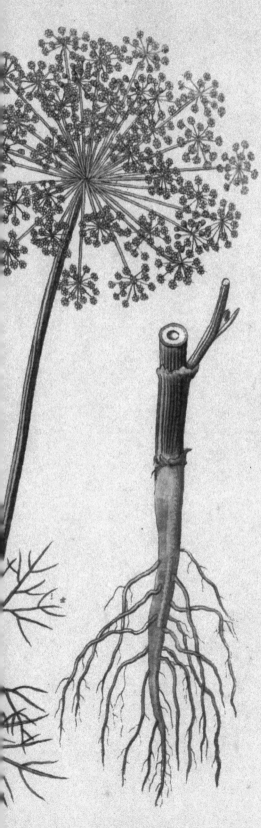

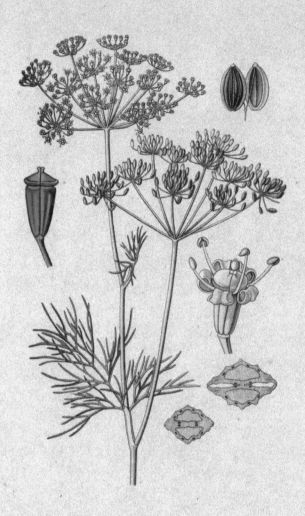

Herbal Magic

Dill is supposed to have been derived from a Norse word to "dull," because the seeds were given to babies to make them sleep. Beyond this innocent employment it was a factor in working spells of the blackest magic.

There is *something* mysterious about it, because, besides being employed in spells by witches and wizards it was used by other people to resist spells cast by traffickers in magic, and was equally powerful to do this.

– Rosalind Northcote, *The Book of Herbs,* **1903**

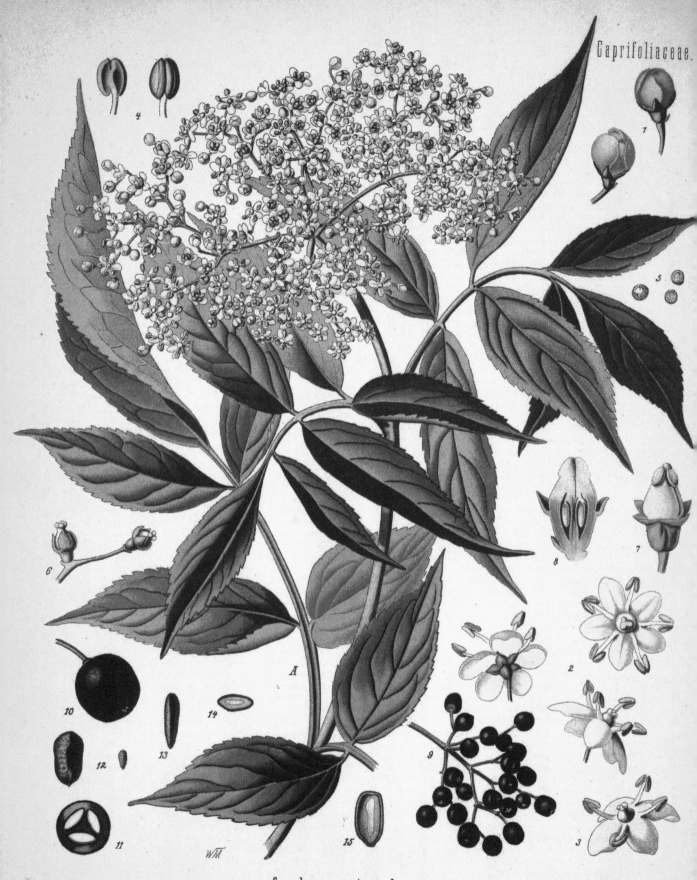

Caprifoliaceae.

Sambucus nigra L.

ELDER

Other Names: Pipe Tree, Bore Tree, Bour Tree,
(Old English) Hylder Eldrum
Latin Name: Sambucus nigra
Symbolises: Zealousness
Type: Deciduous tree or shrub
Natural Habitat: Europe, including Great Britain
Growing Zone: 3–8
Site: Partial shade to full sun
Harvest:
Elder Leaves: April
Elder flowers: June
Elderberries: August to October
Usable Parts: Leaves, flowers, and berries
Companion Plants: Bee balm and flox
Herbal Astrology: Venus

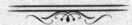

From its pretty white flowers to the legends of witches and magic, the elder tree has been an enduring presence in the rural landscape for centuries. While not a traditional addition to the herb garden, it can be found in shrub, bush, or tree form and boasts an abundance of virtues from its berries to its bark. In parts of England and Scandinavia, the Elder Mother is believed to guard the elder trees. It was said that before taking bark from the elder tree, one would have to ask permission from the Elder Mother, or else bad luck would fall upon them.

The Elder, with its flat-topped masses of creamy-white, fragrant blossoms, followed by large dropping bunches of purplish-black juicy berries, is a familiar object in English countryside and gardens. It has been said, with some truth, that our English summer is not here until the Elder is fully in flower, and that it ends when the elder berries are ripe.

– Maude Grieve, *A Modern Herbal,* **1931**

ELDER

continued.

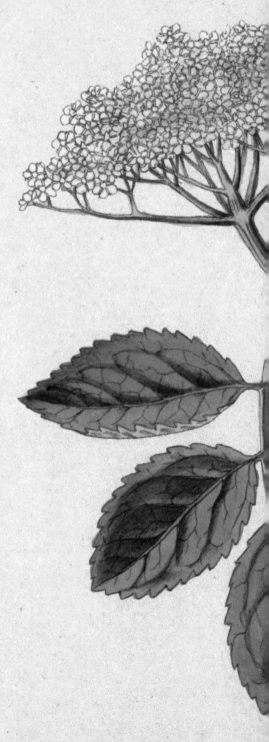

"When elder blossoms bloom upon the bush,
Then women's hearts to sensual pleasure rush."

      – **Charles Godfrey Leland,** *Gypsy Sorcery and Fortune Telling,* **1891**

In the Garden

This succeeds well on a chalky soil, and withstands the smoky
atmosphere of towns. The variety laciniata has deeply-cut leaves,
and aurea is a fine golden-leaved variety. Forms an efficient screen-
fence on poor soil if pruned twice or three times a year.

      – **J. W. Bean,** *Hardy Ornamental Trees and Shrubs,* **1914**

In the Kitchen

Elderflower Lemonade

Put into an earthenware bowl fine, full elder flower blooms, and
for every cluster of flowers pour in 4 quarts of fresh cold water,
add 1 lemon (cut in four), and 2 tablespoonfuls of white vinegar.
Sweeten with 1 1/2lbs. of loaf sugar. Let it stand 24 hours, stirring
occasionally. Then strain and bottle, tying the corks down well. Use
in about 3 weeks.

      – **Various,** *Secrets of Some Wiltshire Housewives,* **1927**

Elderberry Syrup

Cut the berries from the stalk, put them on to simmer, when soft
take them out and squeeze tightly in a cloth. Put the syrup back
into the pan, adding a pound of sugar to a quart of syrup. Cloves
and cayenne to taste. Boil gently until it thickens. Take out when
thick as treacle.

      – **Various,** *Gleanings from Gloucestershire Housewives,* **1936**

ELDER

ANCIENT KNOWLEDGE, VIRTUES, AND LORE

Medicinal Properties and Remedies

The buds of the elder bush, gathered in early spring, and simmered with new butter, or sweet lard, make a very healing and cooling ointment.

— **Lydia Maria Child,** *The American Frugal Housewife,* 1829

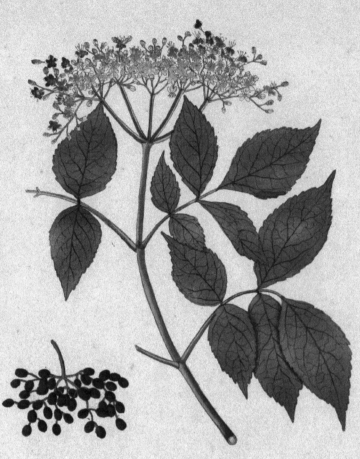

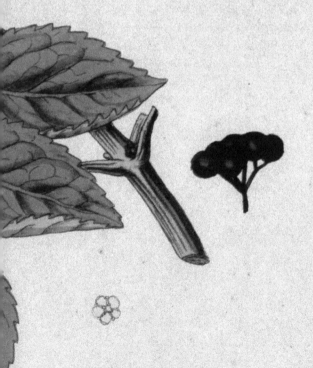

The leaves and young buds are ingredients in many of the teas made for scurvy. The flowers are the chief parts used, which have diaphoretic or sweating powers, discutient, and a fomentation made is good for inflammation. (…) The berries are aperient, the juice of which 2 tablespoonfuls should be taken in fever, rheumatism, arthritic cases, and the exanthemata. Of the powdered bark take 5 grains three times a day for piles. The distilled flowers make a good cooling wash and an excellent mouth water in the morning.

— **Nicholas Culpeper & William Joseph Simmonite,** *Herbal Remedies of Culpeper and Simmonite,* 1957

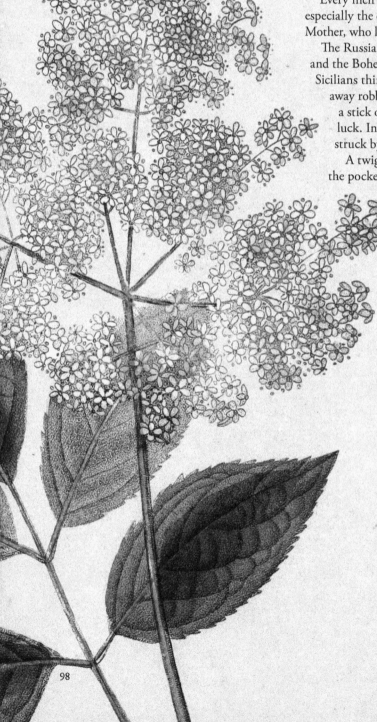

Herbal Magic

Every inch of an Elder-tree is connected with magic. This is especially the case in Denmark. First of all there is the Elder-tree Mother, who lives in the tree and watches for any injury to it. The Russians believe that Elder-trees drive away evil spirits, and the Bohemians go to it, with a spell, to take away fever. The Sicilians think that sticks of its wood will kill serpents and drive away robbers better than any other, and the Serbs introduce a stick of Elder into the wedding ceremonies to bring good luck. In England, it was thought that the Elder was never struck by lightning.

A twig of it tied into three or four knots, and carried in the pocket, was a charm against rheumatism. A cross made of Elder, and fastened to cow-houses and stables, was supposed to keep all evil from the animals.

– Rosalind Northcote, *The Book of Herbs,* **1903**

In order to prevent witches from entering their houses the common people used to gather elder leaves on the last day of April and affix them to their doors and windows.

– Eleanour Sinclair Rohde, *The Old English Herbals,* **1922**

Folk Beliefs

It was said that anyone who accidentally found himself beneath an Elder tree was at once overcome by a great horror and became delirious. The Russian belief, however, is that the Elder tree drives away evil spirits out of compassion to humanity. In Sicily a branch from the Elder tree is considered to be far superior to any other rod for killing serpents and driving away thieves. Scandinavian folklore tells of an Elder tree which once grew in a farmyard and had the unpleasant habit of taking a walk in the twilight and peeping in through the window at the children when they were alone.

– Alexander Porteous, *Forest Folklore, Mythology and Romance,* **1928**

Green elder branches were also buried in a grave to protect the dead from witches and evil spirits, and in some parts it was a custom for the driver of the hearse to carry a whip made of Elder wood.

– Maude Grieve, *A Modern Herbal,* **1931**

In the South of Germany it is believed to drive away evil spirits, and the name "'Holderstock' (Elder Stock) is a term of endearment given by a lover to his beloved, and is connected with Hulda, the old goddess of love, to whom the Elder tree was considered sacred." In Denmark and Norway it is held in like esteem, and in the Tyrol an "Elder bush, trained into the form of a cross, is planted on the new-made grave, and if it blossoms the soul of the person lying beneath it is happy." And this use of the Elder for funeral purposes was, perhaps, also an old English custom; for Spenser, speaking of Death, says—

The Muses that were wont greene Baies to weare,
Now bringen bittre Eldre braunches seare." -

– Henry N. Ellacombe, *The Plant-lore and Garden-craft of Shakespeare,* **1884**

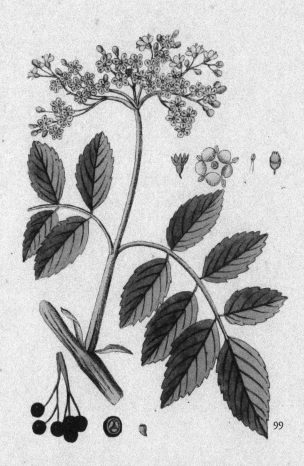

ELDER

continued.

The Legend of the Rollright Stones and the Elder Witch

We must first tell the story as it is most generally told, and which gives as it were the key to many of the others, and to the monument as a whole.

"A certain King, whether Danish or otherwise is not quite sure, landed at Dover, with his army, to invade the country and conquer all England. He there consulted an Oracle or Witch, or Wise woman, all three are mentioned ; who informed him,

"When Long Compton you may see
King of England yon shall be."

Enquiring, he made his way up Rollright hill, marching with his forces until he had nearly reached the top, and at last eager to win the promised crown, hastens in advance of his men and arrives at a spot within a few steps of the crest from which the village of Long Compton would be seen lying in the valley below, when he is met by the Witch of evil eye and horrid shape, to whom the hill belongs, who stops him with the words,

"Seven long strides if thou can'st take,
Take them boldly and win free
If Long Compton thou can'st make,
King of England thou shalt be."

The King who now judged his success assured, cried out exultingly,

"Stand aside; by stick, stock, stone.
As King of England I shall be known!"

He took a stride or two forward, but instead of rising the brow of the hill as he expected, the long mound of earth rose up before him; and before the seven strides were completed, the Witch said,

"Long Compton thou, wilt never see,
King of England thou shalt not be.
Rise up stick and stand still stone,
For King of England thou shalt be none;
Thou and thy men hoar-stones shalt be.
And I myself an eldern-tree.

Whereupon the King, his Army, and the Knights who had lingered behind plotting against him, were all turned into stones as they stood, the King on the side of the mound, his army in a circle behind him, while the Witch herself became an elder tree. But they do say, some day the spell will be broken. The stones will turn again into flesh and blood, and the King will start as an armed warrior at the head of his army to overcome his enemies and rule over the land; while the Witch in vain will try to stop their progress and at last will vanish, to reappear as a spring from out the hill-side. That's how it is that no one dares take away any of the stones; and if they do so, they are bothered out of their lives until they bring them back again.

– **Henry Taunt,** *The Rollright Stones; the Stonehenge of Oxfordshire,* **1888**

ELDER

continued.

Go visit the Rollright on such a night
When the Stones are lit by the pale moonlight.
Softly tread so that none may hear,
Speak not a word—there is naught to fear.

    Thou shalt see
    Fairies wee,
    Elves that ride on the Bumble Bee.
    Pixies free
    Full of glee,
    And a Witch that looks like an Elder Tree.

Yes! The Witch sits there on the altar stone
And cuddles herself and chuckles alone!
Whil'st the wise Owl sits in the fir tree high,
And turns up his eyes to the moon lit sky.

    "To-whit To-woo,
    "What a great to do.
    I'd all go to bed if I were you,
    I never knew
    Such a rowdy crew,
    Or on such a night, such a hullabaloo."

From stone to stone leap the Elfin folk,
Caring nought for the Ravens croak.
Or the White Owls screech or the Banshees cry
Or the Ghosts that over the Circle fly.

    Faster they go
    Above and below,
    Thousands of "Little Folk" to and fro.
    When the East shall glow
    And the cock shall crow,
    Elves and Fairies and Pixies to bed will go.

But go not near that pile of stone,
Where the Whispering Knights for their sins atone.
They were whispering treason too dire to tell,
When the curse of the Witch on them befell,

    So Elf and Fay
    Keep far away
    From the treacherous Knights, who their King
      would slay.
    But blithe and gay
    In the Circle play,
    'Till the Witch sends them home at the break of day.

– **F. C. Rickett,** ***The Rollright Stones, History and Legends***
in Prose and Poetry, **1900**

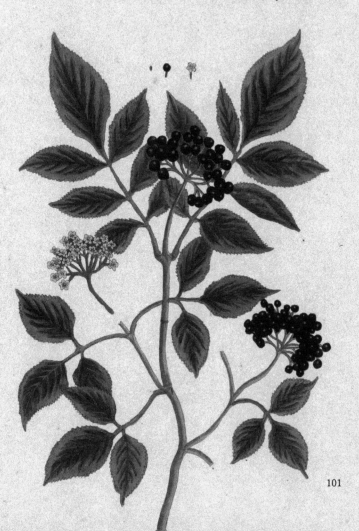

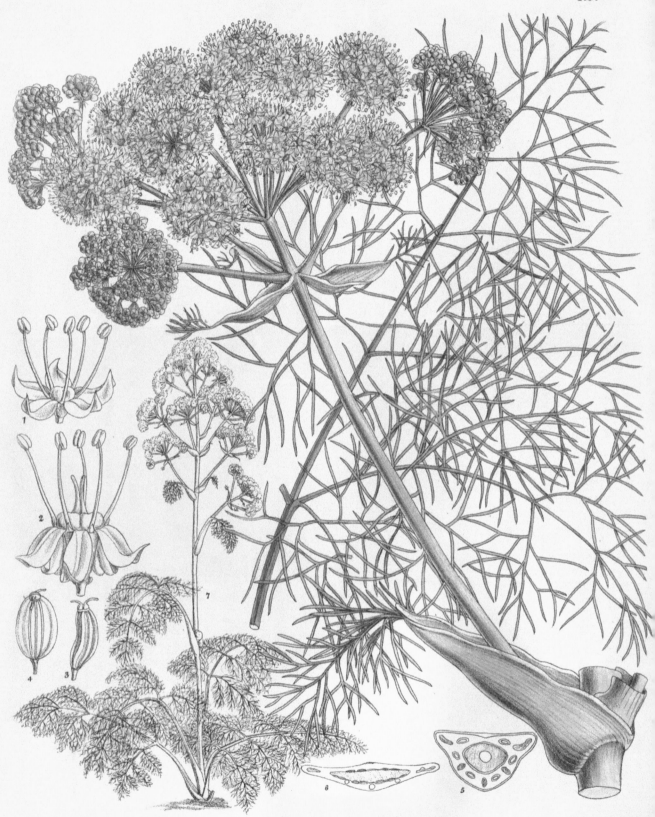

M.S.del.J.N.Fitch lith.

Vincent Brooks,Day&Son,Lt.d imp.

L.Reeve&Cº London

FENNEL

Other Names: **Common Fennel, Sweet Fennel**
Latin Name: **Foeniculum vulgare**
Symbolises: **Worthy all praise, Strength**
Type: **Herbaceous perennial**
Natural Habitat: **Shores of the Mediterranean**
Growing Zone: **4–9**
Site: **Full sun**
Sow: **March to July**
Harvest: **May to October**
Usable Parts: **Leaves, stem, flower, and root**
Companion Plants: **Dill**
Herbal Astrology: **Mercury**

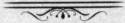

An enchanting herb with airy tops and umbels of yellow flowers, fennel is a versatile ingredient for many dishes in the kitchen. Not to be confused with Florence fennel or finocchio – a variant with the bulb base, often eaten as a vegetable. In Middle Eastern and Indian cooking, its aromatic seeds are used to flavour things such as bread and meat and are a common ingredient in many night-time teas.

COMMON FENNEL (Fœniculum vulgare).—This herb is easily recognized by its leaves, which consist of a number of deeply-divided, hair-like segments, and large terminal umbels of yellow flowers. The whole plant is aromatic, and its chopped leaves are often used as an ingredient in sauce for fish. It grows in waste places, especially near the sea.

– David Ellis, *Medicinal Herbs and Poisonous Plants*, 1918

FENNEL

continued.

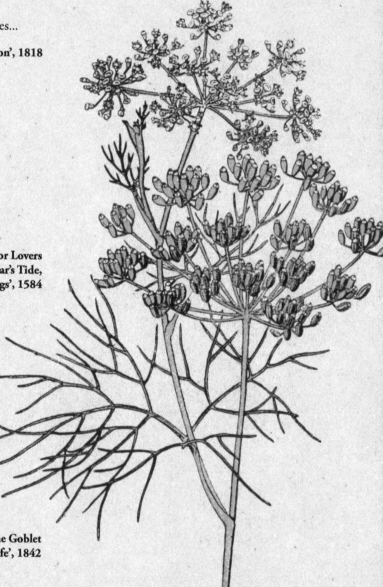

...Be careful, ere ye enter in, to fill
     Your baskets high
With fennel green, and balm, and golden pines...

       – John Keats, 'Endymion', 1818

Fennel is for flaterers,
     an evil thing it is sure:
But I have alwaies meant truely,
     with constant heart most pure;
And will continue in the same
     as long as life doth last,
Still hoping for a ioiful daie,
     when all our paines be past.

   **– William Hunnis, 'A Nosegay Always Sweet, for Lovers
      to Send for Tokens of Love at New Year's Tide,
         or for Fairings', 1584**

Above the lowly plants it towers,
The fennel, with its yellow flowers,
And in an earlier age than ours
Was gifted with the wondrous powers,
   Lost vision to restore.

It gave new strength, and fearless mood;
And gladiators, fierce and rude,
Mingled it in their daily food;
And he who battled and subdued,
   A wreath of Fennel wore.

      **– Henry Wadsworth Longfellow, 'The Goblet
         of Life', 1842**

FENNEL

continued.

In the Garden

Fennel will thrive anywhere, and a plantation will last for years. It is easily propagated by seeds, sown early in April in ordinary soil. It likes plenty of sun and is adapted to dry and sunny situations, not needing heavily manured ground, though it will yield more on rich stiff soil.

— **Maude Grieve,** *A Modern Herbal,* **1931**

"At another spot fennel flourished by itself, as if it had some mysterious power, perhaps its peculiar smell, of keeping other plants at a proper distance. It formed quite a thicket, and grew to a height of ten or twelve feet. This spot was a favourite haunt of mine, as it was in a waste place at the furthest point from the house, a wild solitary spot where I could spend long hours by myself watching the birds. But I also loved the fennel for itself, its beautiful green feathery foliage and the smell of it, also the taste, so that whenever I visited that secluded spot I would rub the crushed leaves in my palms and chew the small twigs for their peculiar fennel flavour."

— **William Henry Hudson,** *Far Away and Long Ago,* **1918**

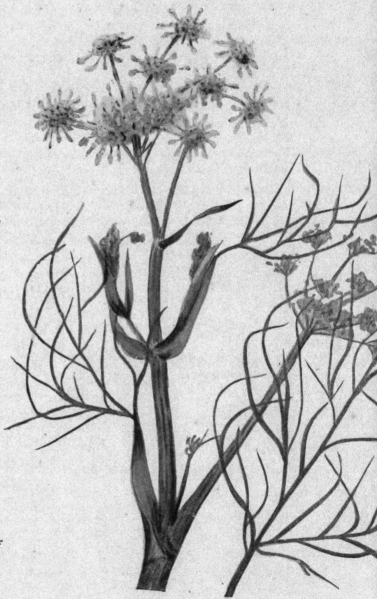

In the Kitchen

In Italy and France, the tender leaves are often used for garnishes and to add flavour to salads, and are also added, finely chopped, to sauces served with puddings. Roman bakers are said to put the herb under their loaves in the oven to make the bread taste agreeably.

FENNEL SAUCE.—Wash and boil green fennel, mint, and parsley, a little of each, till tender; drain and press them, chop them fine and add melted butter; serve up immediately. If the herbs mix long with the butter they will be discoloured.

— **Marcus Woodward,** *The Mistress of Stantons Farm,* **1938**

105

FENNEL

continued.

ANCIENT KNOWLEDGE, VIRTUES, AND LORE

Medicinal Properties and Remedies

Fennel has been rendered famous by the serpent, which tastes it (…) when it casts its old skin, and sharpens its sight with the juice of this plant: a fact which has led to the conclusion that this juice must be beneficial, also, in a high degree to the human sight. Fennel-juice is gathered when the stem is swelling with the bud; after which it is dried in the sun and applied as an ointment with honey. This plant is to be found in all parts of the world. The most esteemed preparation from it, is that made in Iberia, from the tear-like drops which exude from the stalk and the seed fresh-gathered. The juice is extracted, also, from incisions made in the root at the first germination of the plant.

> – **Elder Pliny**, *The Natural History of Pliny*, c. 77 AD

Fennel Water

It may be made by rubbing oil with carbonate of magnesia; adding water, and filtering through paper, as in the case of cinnamon water. Boiling water, however, extracts the essential properties, and *Fennel tea* is a common preparation as a domestic carminative.

> – **Robley Dunglison**, *General Therapeutics and Materia Medica*, 1850

The infusion, prepared by adding two or three drams of the seeds to boiling water, is the best form for administering it.

> – **George Ripley**, *American Cyclopaedia*, 1881

Herbal Magic

Traditionally the fennel shares with Saint John's wort, the houseleek and stone crop the magic virtue of protecting a house from evil influences and from fire, and sprigs of fennel are carried as amulets still in some parts of the country.

> – **Mary Thorne Quelch**, *A Guide to your Herb Garden*, 1951

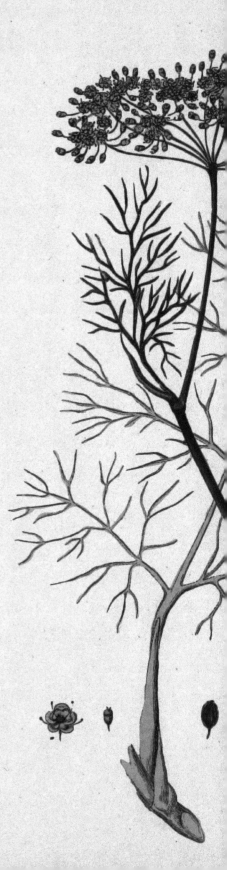

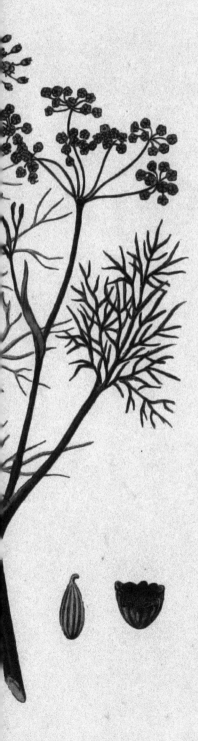

Folk Beliefs

In Shakespeare's time we have the plainest evidence that it was the recognized emblem of flattery (…) it's said that Ophelia's flowers were all chosen for their significance, so, perhaps, it was not by accident that she offers fennel to her brother, in whose ears the cry must have been still ringing,

"choose we; Laertes shall be king!"

– Rosalind Northcote, *The Book of Herbs,* **1903**

As far back as the time of Pliny serpents were supposed to be very fond of fennel, restoring to them their youth by enabling them to cast their old skins.

– Thomas Firminger Thistelton-Dyer, *Folk-lore of Plants,* **1889**

The Greek name for fennel is *marathon.* The Battle of Marathon took its name from the plant. The story goes that a youth named Pheidippides ran to Sparta to seek aid for Athens when the Persian fleet appeared, and he was told that the Spartans could not come until the full moon. Very disheartened, he was returning to Athens when Pan appeared to him and promised victory, giving the youth a piece of fennel as a token of his prophecy. The battle took place on a field full of fennel and was known henceforth as the Battle of Marathon (490 B.C.). Statues of the youth always represented him as holding a sprig of fennel.

– Esther Singleton, *The Shakespeare Garden,* **1922**

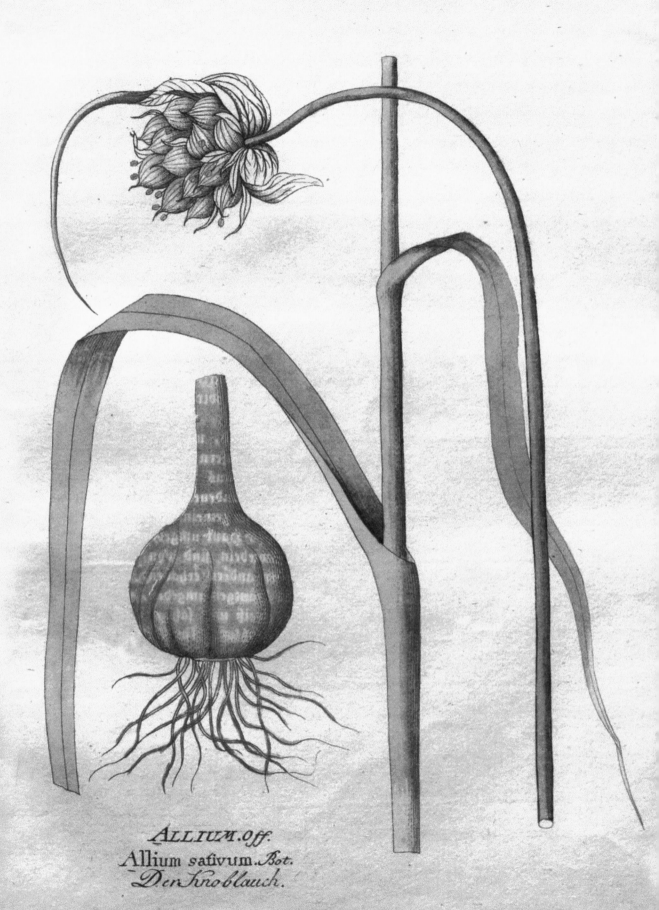

Allium. off.

Allium sativum. *Bot.*

Der Knoblauch.

GARLIC

Other Names: Poor Man's Treacle, Stinking Rose,
Camphor of the Poor, Russian Penicillin
Latin Name: Allium sativum
Symbolises: Strength and courage
Type: Annual
Natural Habitat: Central Asia
Growing Zone: 1–5
Site: Full sun
Sow: October to February
Harvest: June to August
Usable Parts: Bulb, leaves, stem, and flowers
Companion Plants: Chamomile, dill, and nasturtiums,
Herbal Astrology: Mars

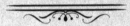

Garlic's diverse medicinal properties have bolstered human health for centuries, from calming inflammatory diseases to preventing the common cold. Despite the bulb being used the most in cooking, the scapes (the tender stem and flower buds) can be deliciously whizzed into pesto or sauteed among other green vegetables.

The Common Garlic a member of the same group of plants as the Onion, is of such antiquity as a cultivated plant, that it is difficult with any certainty to trace the country of its origin. De Candolle, in his treatise on the Origin of Cultivated Plants, considered that it was apparently indigenous to the southwest of Siberia, whence it spread to southern Europe, where it has become naturalized, and is said to be found wild in Sicily. It is widely cultivated in the Latin countries bordering on the Mediterranean. Dumas has described the air of Provence as being 'particularly perfumed by the refined essence of this mystically attractive bulb.'

– Maude Grieve, *A Modern Herbal,* **1931**

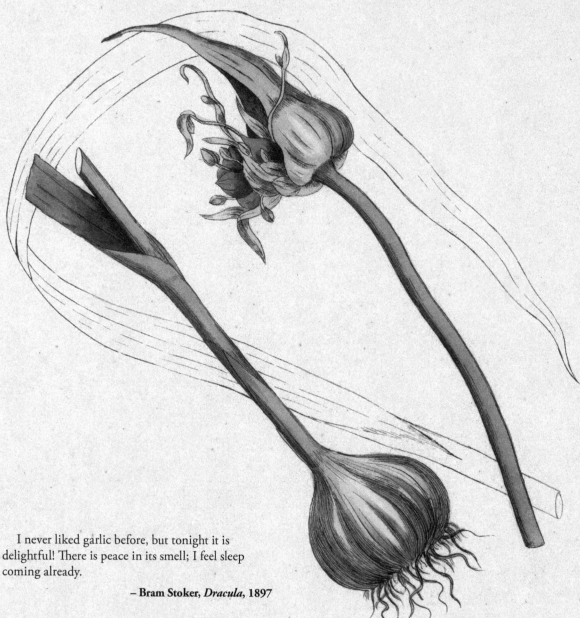

I never liked garlic before, but tonight it is delightful! There is peace in its smell; I feel sleep coming already.

– Bram Stoker, *Dracula,* **1897**

– I had rather live
With cheese and garlic in a windmill, far,
Than feed on cates and have him talk to me
In any summerhouse in Christendom.

– William Shakespeare, *King Henry IV,*
Act 3, Scene 1, 1597

…No! you won't 'eed nothin' else
But them spicy garlic smells,
An' the sunshine an' the palm-trees an' the tinkly
  temple-bells;…

– Rudyard Kipling, 'Mandalay', 1890

GARLIC

continued.

In the Garden

The same kind of soils which are suitable for the growth of onions is adapted to garlic. Some merely press the cloves with the fingers and thumb upon a finely-prepared soft surface, and cover them over with a little earth. They should be hoed and weeded in the same manner as onions, and the ground kept perfectly clear during the summer.

Put into the ground as early as October; but if, from any cause, the planting is deferred, they will answer if sown in February or March. Garlic throws up a stem bearing at the top a bunch of small bulbs enclosed in a kind of sheath. As this takes away the strength which would otherwise be directed to the bulb, gardeners usually tie the stem and leaves into a knot, as they approach maturity, to check this development.

– Isabella Beeton, *Gardening,* **1861**

It deserves a place in the herb garden, not only because of its classical associations, but because in flower it is so decorative. Garlic does best in a rich but well-drained soil and in full sun. There are about ten cloves to each bulb and the cloves should be planted separately about two inches deep and six inches apart.

– Eleanour Sinclair Rohde, *Herbs and Herb Gardening,* **1936**

Garlic is dug up... from cultivated plants when the leaves begin to wither, and with a portion of the flowering stem attached; the bulbs are then cleaned and after being dried in the sun they are tied in bunches, and thus brought into the market. They are said to lose in drying nine parts of their weight, but with little loss of their sensible properties. They are best preserved by hanging them up in a dry place.

– Robert Bentley, *Medicinal Plants,* **1880**

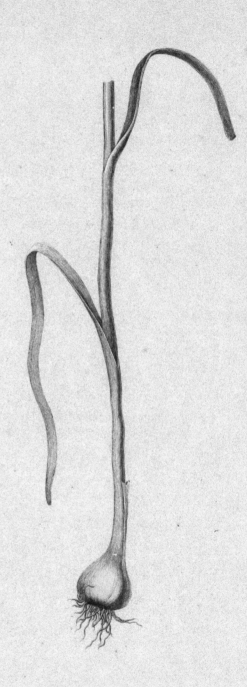

GARLIC

In the Kitchen

It is used in many preparations, but can be omitted and replaced by using shallots or onions, when desired. Garlic, when used in salad, should be rubbed on a crust of bread (called chapon). When used for stews, etc., and left whole, its flavor will not be strong and penetrating as when mashed or chopped, and gives the preparation an appetizing and agreeable taste, especially in mutton stews.

— **Jules Arthur Harder,** *The Physiology of Taste,* **1885**

If garlic or onions are wanted to keep some time, the heads should be dipped in salt water, made lukewarm; by doing this, they will be all the better for keeping, though quite worthless for reproduction. Some persons content themselves with hanging them over burning coals, and are of opinion that this is quite sufficient to prevent them from sprouting: for it is a well-known fact, that both garlic and onions sprout when out of the ground, and that after throwing out their thin shoots they shrivel away to nothing. Some persons are of opinion, too, that the best way of keeping garlic is by storing it in chaff.

— **Elder Pliny,** *The Natural History of Pliny,* **c. 77 AD**

GARLIC VINEGAR

1 bunch garlic
1 bottle vinegar

1. Peel the cloves of garlic, then put them through a food chopper into a bowl.
2. Put this pulp and juice into a bottle of vinegar, cork and leave for two weeks, then strain.

This vinegar is delicious in salad dressings for all kinds of fish.

— **Marion Neil Harris,** *Beverages, Vinegars, and Syrups,* **1914**

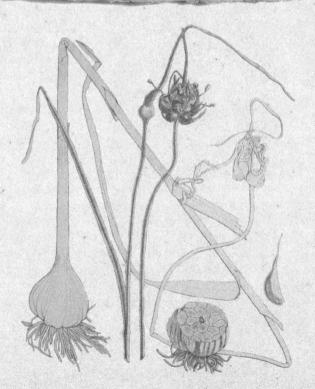

GARLIC

continued.

ANCIENT KNOWLEDGE, VIRTUES, AND LORE

Medicinal Properties and Remedies

Like onions, chives and shallots, it possesses medicinal virtues, being cooling to the system, increasing saliva and gastric juices, stimulating, and digestive.

– Charles Herman Senn, *Senn's Culinary Encyclopaedia,* **1898**

As an antiseptic, its use has long been recognized. In the late war it was widely employed in the control of suppuration in wounds. The raw juice is expressed, diluted with water, and put on swabs of sterilized Sphagnum moss, which are applied to the wound. Where this treatment has been given, it has been proved that there have been no septic results, and the lives of thousands of men have been saved by its use.

– Maude Grieve, *A Modern Herbal,* **1931**

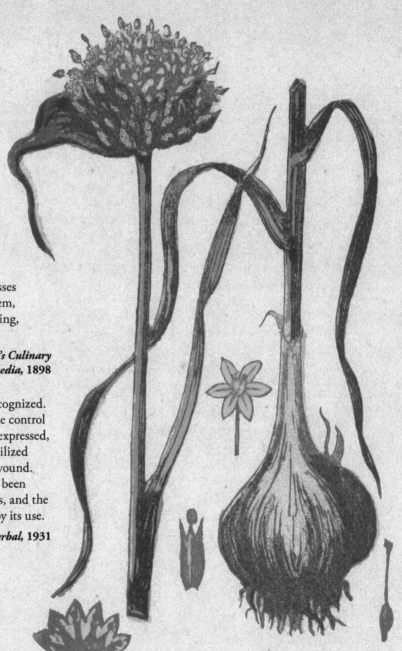

Herbal Magic

We find in many forms spread far and wide the belief that garlic possesses the magic power of protection against poison and sorcery. This comes, according to Pliny, from the fact that when it is hung up in the open air for a time, it turns black, when it is supposed to attract evil into itself—and, consequently, to withdraw it from the wearer. The ancients believed that the herb which Mercury gave to Ulysses to protect him from the enchantment of Circe, and which Homer calls moly, was the alium nigrum, or garlic, the poison of the witch being a narcotic. Among the modern Greeks and Turks, garlic is regarded as the most powerful charm against evil spirits, magic, and misfortune. For this reason they carry it with them, and hang it up in their houses as a protection against storms and bad weather. So their sailors carry with them a sack of it to avert shipwreck. If anyone utters a word of praise with the intention of fascinating or of doing harm, they cry aloud 'Garlic!' or utter it three times rapidly.

– **Charles Godfrey Leland,** *Gypsy Sorcery and Fortune Telling,* **1891**

To dream of eating garlic shows that you will find it possible to put up with the vexations and vicissitudes of life in an astonishingly cheerful manner; to be picking it means that you desire to come to the root of some matter of which at present you have only an inkling: if the garlic comes up by the root as you pick it, you will discover the secret: if it breaks off in your hand, it will remain a mystery.

– **Madame Juno,** *Gypsy Queen Dream Book and Fortune Teller,* **1930**

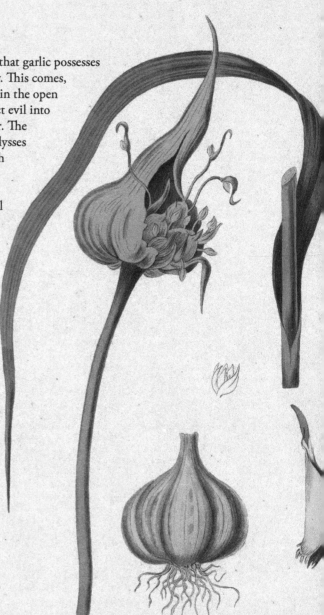

GARLIC

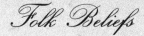

Folk Beliefs

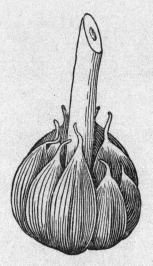

For the purpose of depriving all these plants of their strong smell, it is recommended to set them when the moon is below the horizon, and to take them up when she is in conjunction.

– Elder Pliny, *The Natural History of Pliny,* **c. 77 AD**

[Garlic] formed the principal ingredient in the 'Four Thieves' Vinegar,' which was adapted so successfully at Marseilles for protection against the plague when it prevailed there in 1722. This originated, it is said, with four thieves who confessed, that whilst protected by the liberal use of aromatic vinegar during the plague, they plundered the dead bodies of its victims with complete security.

(…)

There is a curious superstition in some parts of Europe, that if a morsel of the bulb be chewed by a man running a race it will prevent his competitors from getting ahead of him, and Hungarian jockeys will sometimes fasten a clove of Garlic to the bits of their horses in the belief that any other racers running close to those thus baited, will fall back the instant they smell the offensive odour.

– Maude Grieve, *A Modern Herbal,* **1931**

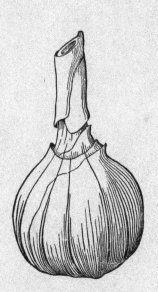

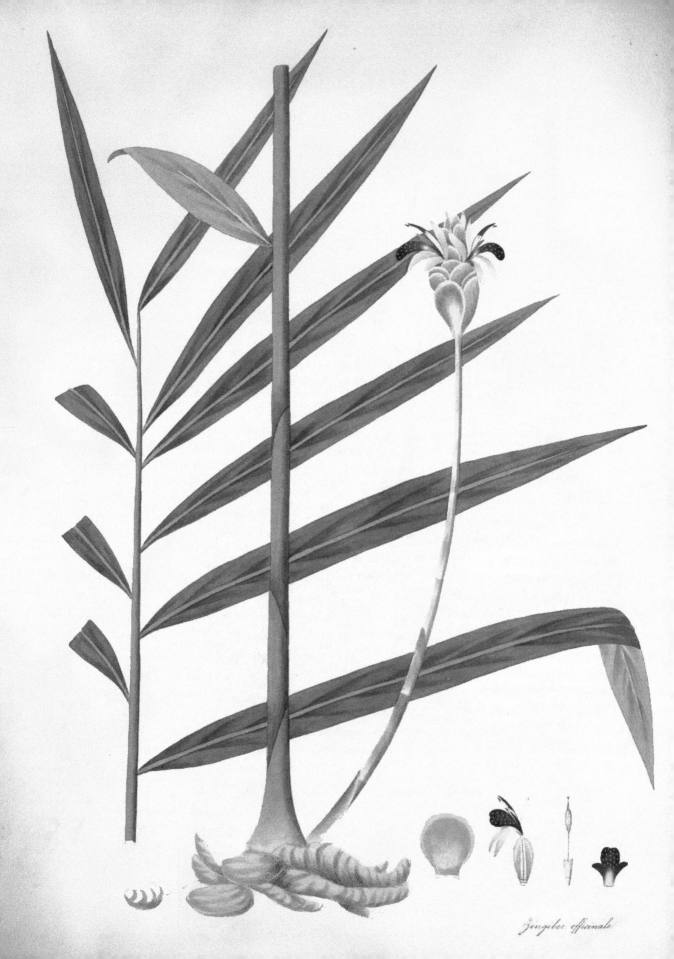

Zingiber officinale

GINGER

Other Names: Ginger Root
Latin Name: Zingiber officinale
Symbolises: Fiery passion
Type: Tender Herbaceous perennial
Natural Habitat: Cultivated in West Indies, Jamaica, Africa
Growing Zone: 9–12
Site: Warm and sheltered spot. Best grown indoors
in pots in cooler zones
Sow: March
Harvest: Ten months after planting
Usable Parts: Root
Companion Plants: Chillis, coriander, garlic, and leafy greens
Herbal Astrology: Mars

Now primarily associated with coughs and colds, the spiced root of ginger boasts a warming quality and has been used in folk medicine for centuries. While an untraditional addition to the herb garden, it is surprisingly easy to grow in pots as long as it is kept in a warm and sheltered spot while the roots and shoots develop.

Ginger is an aromatic plant, a native of Hindostan, and is cultivated in all parts of India and China. The root is the portion in which the virtues of the plant reside. After the roots are gathered and cleansed they are scalded in boiling water, to prevent germination, and are then rapidly dried. This is the ordinary black ginger, most of which comes from Calcutta, and is called East India Ginger. In Jamaica another variety is prepared by selecting the best roots, depriving them of their epidermis and drying them carefully in the sun. This is the highly valued white Ginger, generally called Jamaica Ginger. A preserve is made from Ginger by selecting the young roots, depriving them of their cortical covering and boiling them in syrup. This is imported from the East and West Indies, and from China. When good it is translucent and tender. The odor of Ginger is aromatic and penetrating, the taste spicy, pungent, hot, and biting. These properties gradually diminish and are ultimately lost by exposure. It is used by pastry cooks, and confectioners, in putting up spiced preserves and fruits. Ginger is a grateful stimulant and carminative, and is often given in dyspepsia, flatulent colic, and the feeble state of the alimentary canal attendant upon atonic gout.

– Jules Arthur Harder, *The Physiology of Taste*, 1885

Nose, nose, jolly red nose,
And what gave thee thy jolly red nose?
Nutmeg and ginger, cinnamon and cloves:
That's what gave me this jolly red nose.

–Thomas Ravenscroft, 'Of All the Birds', 1609

In the Garden

The herbaceous part of the plant withers in December, and the roots are dug up in January; but when the root is intended to be preserved in syrup, it is dug up when the shoots do not exceed five or six inches in height. For preparing the dried ginger, after the roots are dug, the best pieces are selected, scraped, then washed, and dried in the sun with great care.

– Anthony Todd Thomson, *The London Dispensatory*, 1811

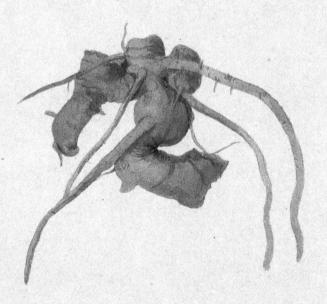

In the Kitchen

Eliza Acton's Gingerbread, 1845

Ingredients:

Eggs 5
Treacle 1 1/4 lb.
Pale brown sugar 6 oz.
Flour 1 lb.
Butter 6 oz. (not margarine)
Ground ginger 1 oz.
Lemons, grated rind of 2.

Time: to bake, about 2 hours.

Method:

1. Beat eggs well.

2. Add warmed syrup gradually, beating all the time.

3. Add sugar in same manner.

4. Add butter, which must be warmed but not hot.

5. Add the ginger to the flour and sift the two together. Add to egg mixture.

6. Beat till bubbles appear in batter, then add flavouring.

7. Bake in greased shallow tin in slow oven.

– Florence White, *Good Things in England – A Practical Cookery*, 1932

GINGER

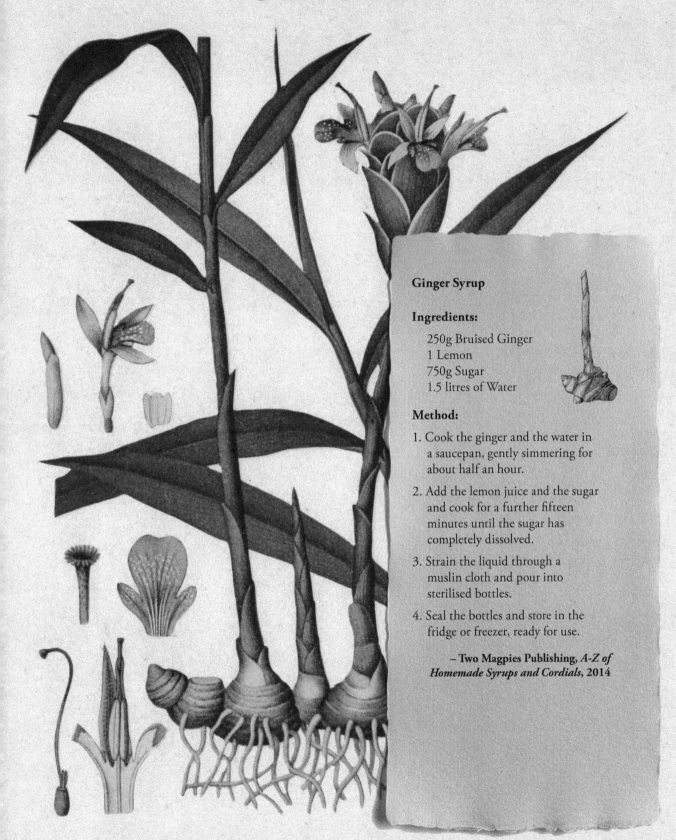

Ginger Syrup

Ingredients:

250g Bruised Ginger
1 Lemon
750g Sugar
1.5 litres of Water

Method:

1. Cook the ginger and the water in a saucepan, gently simmering for about half an hour.

2. Add the lemon juice and the sugar and cook for a further fifteen minutes until the sugar has completely dissolved.

3. Strain the liquid through a muslin cloth and pour into sterilised bottles.

4. Seal the bottles and store in the fridge or freezer, ready for use.

– **Two Magpies Publishing,** *A-Z of Homemade Syrups and Cordials,* **2014**

GINGER

continued.

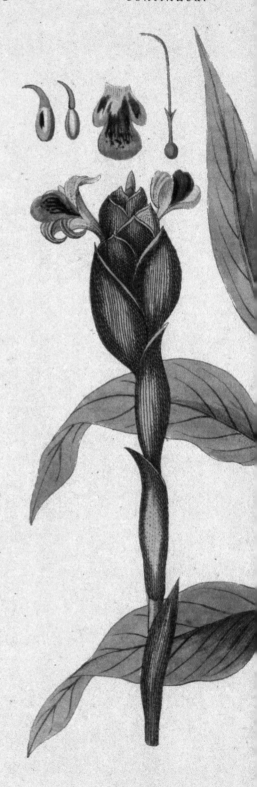

ANCIENT KNOWLEDGE, VIRTUES, AND LORE

Medicinal Properties and Remedies

The stimulating, aromatic, and carminative properties render it of much value in atonic dyspepsia, especially if accompanied with much flatulence; and as an adjunct to purgative medicines to correct griping. When chewed it is frequently serviceable in relaxed conditions of the uvula and tonsils. As a rubefacient it will frequently relieve headache and toothache.

— **Robert Bentley,** *Medicinal Plants,* **1880**

Helps digestion, warms the stomach, clears the sight, and is profitable for old men: heats the joints, and therefore is profitable against the gout, expels wind; it is hot and dry in the second degree.

— **Nicholas Culpeper,** *Complete Herbal,* **1824**

GINGER

continued.

Folk Beliefs

Ginger was known to the Romans, and is said by Pliny to have been brought from Arabia. (French Gingerbread) Pain d'épice, made of rye-flour, honey, ginger, and other spices, was sold in Paris as early as the 14th century. It was probably introduced into England in the reign of Henry the Fourth, and shortly afterwards treacle was used in making it, instead of honey. Gingerbread made with treacle being darker than that made with honey, it was covered with gold-leaf or gilt paper to disguise its colour; hence arose our familiar proverb about taking "the gilt off the gingerbread."

– **Charles Herman Senn,** *A Pocket Dictionary of Foods &*
Culinary Encyclopaedia, **1908**

The Motu (Papuasian) were accustomed to rub spears with ginger to make them fly straight.

– **Carveth Read,** *The Origin of Man and of His Superstitions,* **1920**

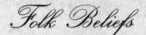

121

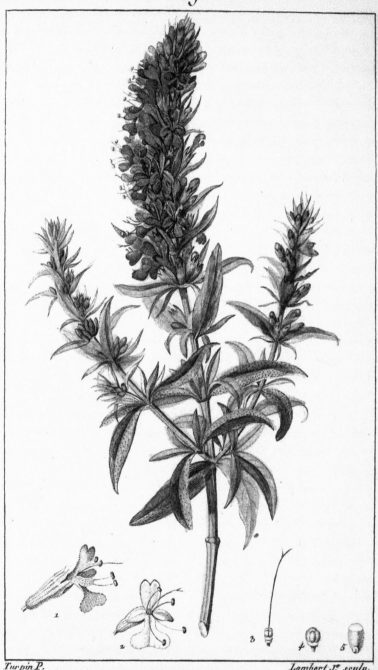

Turpin P.

Lambert J.e sculp.

HYSSOPE.

a.l.l.

HYSSOP

Other Names: Herbe de Joseph, Hissopo
Latin Name: Hyssopus officinalis
Symbolises: Cleanliness
Type: Semi-evergreen perennial
Natural Habitat: Southern Europe
Growing Zone: 4–9
Site: Full sun, moist but well-drained soil
Sow: March to April
Harvest: Four weeks after planting
Usable Parts: Flowering tops and leaves
Companion Plants: Catmint, chives, garlic, lavender, and rosemary
Herbal Astrology: Jupiter

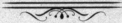

Belonging to the mint family, hyssop has been grown in herb gardens since the Middle Ages, when it was a popular ingredient for stuffings and soups. No longer as popular now, this lofty herb with its delicate purple blooms is primarily used to give absinthe its distinct green colour. The leaves can also be made into a floral but calming tea, much like those made from lavender buds.

Hyssop is a pleasant old-fashioned evergreen shrub formerly grown in every garden. Its uses were manifold. Mazes were set out with Hyssop, the leaves were used in salads and broths, a decoction of the herb was a common remedy for chest complaints and the golden Hyssop Parkinson describes as "of so pleasant a colour, that it provoked every gentlewoman to wear it on their heads and on their arms with as much delight as any fine flowers can give".

– Eleanour Sinclair Rohde, *Herbs and Herb Gardening,* **1936**

HYSSOP

continued.

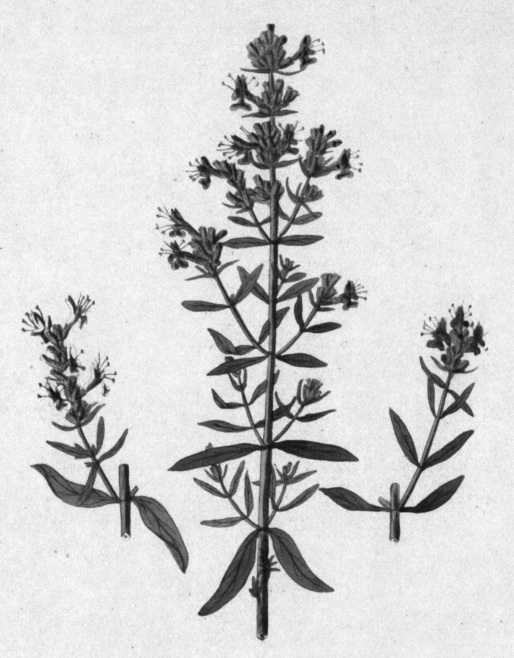

Our bodies are our gardeners; so that if we will
plant nettles, or sow lettuce, set hyssop and weed up
thyme (...) why the power and corrigible authority of
this lies in our wills.

– William Shakespeare, *Othello*, **Act 1, Scene 3, 1604**

HYSSOP

continued.

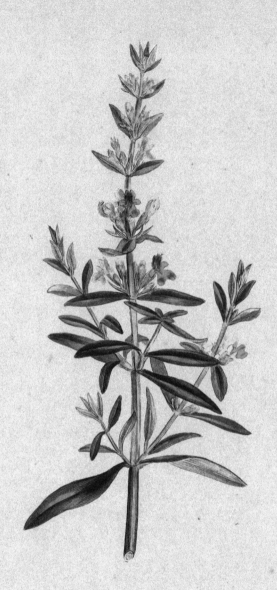

In the Garden

Hyssop should be sowed in March or April; rooted off-sets may be taken in these months or in August and September, or cuttings from the stems in April or May, and these should be watered two or three times a week till they have struck. Both Hyssop and Sage are the better for being cut back when they have finished flowering.

— **Rosalind Northcote**, *The Book of Herbs*, 1903

Sow them in a dry, sandy soil, and thin them out to eight inches apart.

— **Jules Arthur Harder**, *The Physiology of Taste*, 1885

In common with most natives of Southern Europe Hyssop likes a light soil and full sun. It is easily raised from seed or cuttings. Left unclipped Hyssop makes rather an untidy shrub between two and three feet high and nearly as much across. It takes kindly to clipping but this sacrifices the flowers.

— **Eleanour Sinclair Rohde**, *Herbs and Herb Gardening*, 1936

In the Kitchen

Hyssop was used both in cookery and medicine even in our grandmother's days. The young tops and flowers were used to flavour pottage, they were a common ingredient in salads, and hyssop tea and syrup were accounted excellent cordials. An old receipt book recommends hyssop in warm ale, taken fasting in the morning, 'to cause an excellent colour and complexion.'

— **Eleanour Sinclair Rohde**, *The Scented Garden*, 1900

HYSSOP

continued.

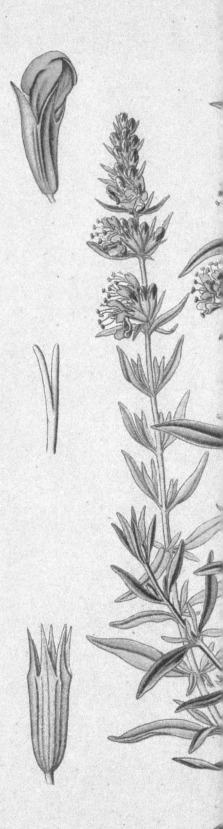

ANCIENT KNOWLEDGE, VIRTUES, AND LORE

Medicinal Properties and Remedies

Stimulant, aromatic, carminative, and tonic. Generally used in quinsy and other sore-throats, as a gargle with sage. As an expectorant it is beneficial in asthma, coughs, etc. The leaves applied to bruises speedily relieve the pain and remove the discolouration.

> **– Oliver Phelps Brown,** *The Complete Herbalist,* **1885**

Hyssop Tea.
Pour one pint of boiling water on one dram of the green tops.

A Water to cause an Excellent Colour and Complexion.
Drink six spoonfuls of the juice of Hyssop in warm Ale in a Morning and fasting. — From *The Receipt Book of John Nott*, Cook to the Duke of Bolton, 1723.

To make Syrup of Hysop for Colds.
Take an handful of Hysop, of Figs, Raysins, Dates, of each an ounce, French Barley one ounce, boyl therein three pintes of fair water to a quart, strain it and clarifie it with two Whites of Eggs, then put in two pound of fine Sugar and boyl it to a Syrup. — From *The Queen's Closet Opened*, by W. M., Cook to Queen Henrietta Maria, 1655

HYSSOP

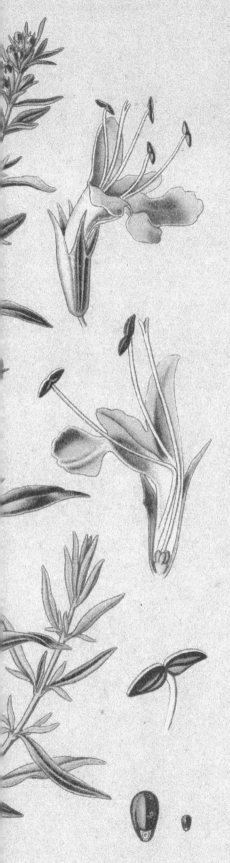

– Eleanour Sinclair Rohde, *A Garden of Herbs,* **1921**

It is an excellent medicine for the quinsy, or swellings in the throat, to wash and gargle it, being boiled in figs; it helps the toothache, being boiled in vinegar and gargled therewith. The hot vapours of the decoction taken by a funnel in at the ears, eases the inflammations and singing noise of them. Being bruised, and salt, honey, and cummin seed put to it, helps those that are stung by serpents. The oil thereof (the head being anointed) kills lice, and takes away itching of the head. It helps those that have the falling sickness, which way soever it be applied…The green herb bruised and a little sugar put hereto, doth quickly heal any cut or green wounds, being thereunto applied.

– Nicholas Culpeper, *Complete Herbal,* **1824**

Herbal Magic

As a protection against the Evil Eye, [hyssop] was hung up in houses.

– Rosalind Northcote, *The Book of Herbs,* **1903**

Folk Beliefs

Hyssop is a name of Greek origin. The Hyssopos of Dioscorides was named from azob (a holy herb), because it was used for cleaning sacred places. It is alluded to in the Scriptures: 'Purge me with Hyssop, and I shall be clean.'

– Maude Grieve, *A Modern Herbal,* **1931**

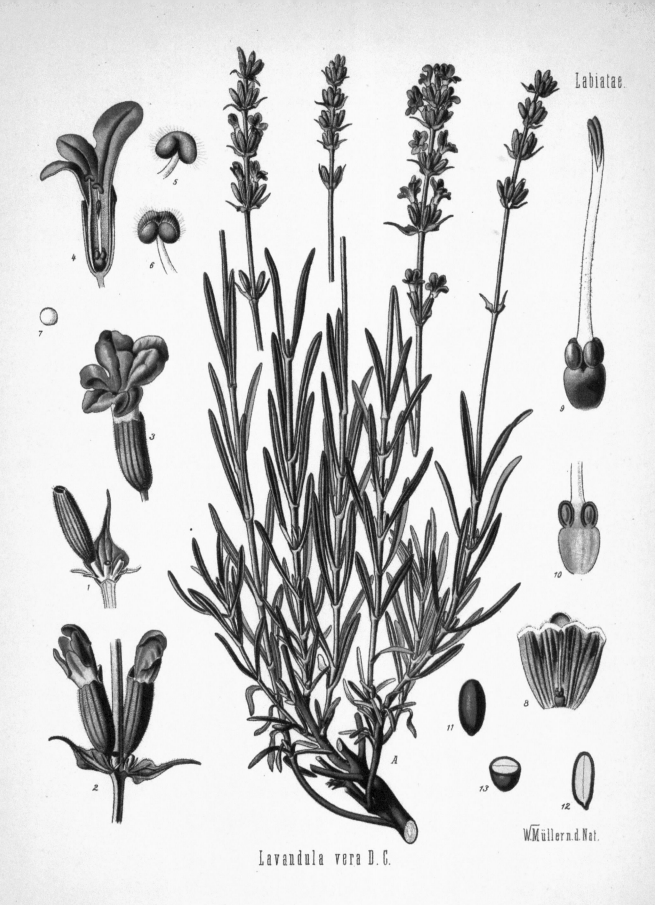

Labiatae.

Lavandula vera D.C.

W.Müller n.d.Nat.

LAVENDER

Other Names: English Lavender, Spike Lavender, True Lavender
Latin Name: Lavandula angustifolia
Symbolises: Distrust
Type: Herbaceous perennial
Natural Habitat: Shores of the Mediterranean
Growing Zone: 5–9
Site: Full sun
Sow: April to May, or October
Harvest: Best picked early in the morning
Usable Parts: Flowering tops
Companion Plants: Echinacea, marigolds, sage, rosemary, and roses
Herbal Astrology: Mercury

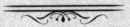

An essential herb for insomniacs, lavender's enchanting scent is used abundantly in pillow mists, candles, and teas for those seeking a blissful night's sleep. Traditionally, its distinctive scent was more commonly used to keep homes and clothes fragrant, with dried sprigs placed between freshly laundered sheets. To harvest lavender for drying, pick the stems in the early spring before all the buds have come into flower.

A native of the south of Europe, the plant was introduced to England in the sixteenth century, but probably was still rare in the Elizabethan era, though mentioned by Spenser as "the Lavender still gray," and by Gerard as growing in his garden: it was not put by Bacon in his list of sweet-smelling plants. All parts of the shrub give out the aromatic odour, recalling, besides inns, old-world gardens, with belles and beaux taking the air.

Lavender is ever associated with all things clean, fresh and of good repute, and we recall that the name is from Lavendula, and that the old form of our "laundress" was "a Lavendre."

– Marcus Woodward, *How to Enjoy Flowers*, 1928

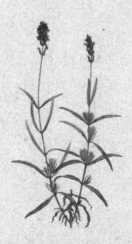

LAVENDER

continued.

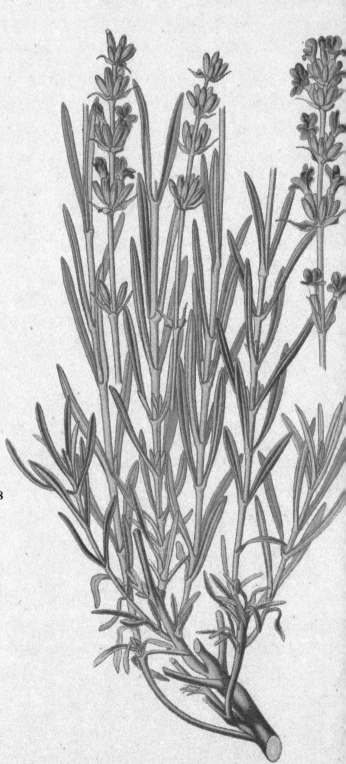

Gray walls that lichen stains,
That take the sun and the rains,
   Old, stately, and wise:
Clipt yews, old lawns flag-bordered,
In ancient ways yet ordered;
   South walks where the loud bee plies
   Daylong till Summer flies —
Here grows Lavender, here breathes England.

Gay cottage gardens, glad,
Comely, unkempt, and mad,
   Jumbled, jolly, and quaint;
Nooks where some old man dozes;
Currants and beans and roses
   Mingling without restraint;
   A wicket that long lacks paint —
Here grows Lavender, here breathes England.

Sprawling for elbow-room,
Spearing straight spikes of bloom,
   Clean, wayward, and tough;
Sweet and tall and slender,
True, enduring, and tender,
   Buoyant and bold and bluff,
   Simplest, sanest of stuff —
Thus grows Lavender, thence breathes England.

      – **W. W. Blair Fish, 'Lavender', 1918**

LAVENDER

In the Garden

To secure really first-rate Lavender not only must the ground be thoroughly dug to a depth of three feet before planting but the soil round the bushes has to be kept well hoed and as near the main stem as possible. It is curious how frequently Lavender is neglected in this respect.

Lavender is usually increased by cuttings, choosing young growths about six inches long. Commercial growers now take very small cuttings less than three inches long, as plants raised thus are less liable to Shab disease. In gardens the cuttings can be set six inches apart and transplanted when well rooted and large enough to handle. Early spring or October are suitable times. Deep planting is essential. The plants should be put in leaving barely two inches of stem above ground and the soil round made very firm.

– Eleanour Sinclair Rohde, *Herbs and Herb Gardening,* **1936**

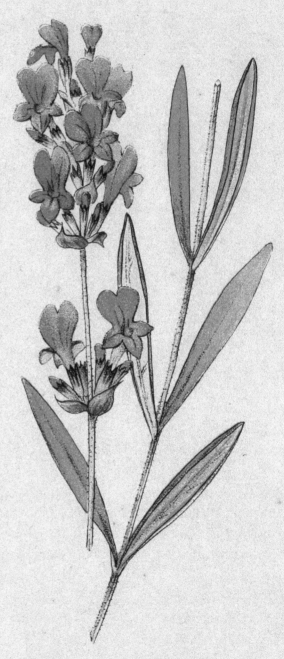

These all flower about the end of June, and beginning of July, and although *Clusius* saith he found the last about *Malaca* in flower in February, and in March about *Murcia,* yet it doth not flower in these colder Countries until June at the soonest, or July.

– John Parkinson, *Theatrum Botanicum: The Theater of Plants,* **1640**

The flowers are picked when the lower-most ones have just appeared; they are stripped from the stalk and dried. The oil-glands are chiefly confined to the calyx, and appear on this structure (itself bluish-violet) as shining bodies, easily visible with the help of a pocket-lens.

– David Ellis, *Medicinal Herbs and Poisonous Plants,* **1918**

Lavender has been unusually fine; to reap its fragrant harvest is one of the many joys of the flower year. If it is to be kept and dried, it should be cut when as yet only a few of the purple blooms are out on the spike; if left too late, the flower shakes off the stalk too readily.

– Henry Wadsworth Longfellow, *The Complete Poetical Works of Henry Wadsworth Longfellow,* **1851**

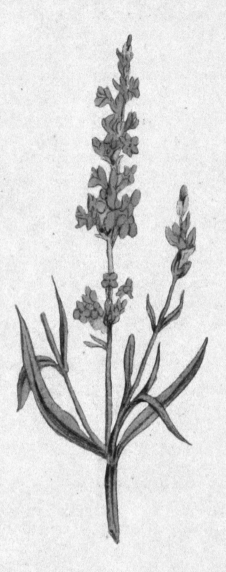

In the Kitchen

Lavender was used in earlier days as a condiment and for flavouring dishes 'to comfort the stomach.' Gerard speaks of Conserves of Lavender being served at table.

– Maude Grieve, *A Modern Herbal,* **1931**

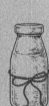

Lavender Flower Syrup

Ingredients

100g Lavender Flowers
500ml Boiling Water
400g Sugar (or partly replace with 200g honey)

Method

1. Place the flowers into a large jar or bowl and pour the boiling water over them.

2. Cover with a clean cloth and leave to stand until cool.

3. Pour the mixture into a heavy-bottomed saucepan with the sugar / honey and boil for ten minutes.

4. Strain the mixture through a clean muslin cloth and pour into sterilised bottles to store.

– Two Magpies Publishing, *The A-Z of Homemade Jams and Jellies,* **2013**

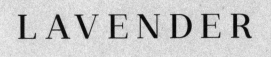

LAVENDER

continued.

ANCIENT KNOWLEDGE, VIRTUES, AND LORE

Medicinal Properties and Remedies

The medicinal virtues of lavender reside entirely in its essential oil, which experience proves to be a gentle stimulant of the aromatic kind. Dr. Cullen observes, that among the plants entitled cephalics, lavender has perhaps the best title to it; and whether applied externally, or given internally, it is a powerful stimulant to the nervous system.

– **George Spratt,** *Flora Medica,* **1829**

The oil for cold and benumbed parts and is almost wholly spent with us for to perfume linen, apparel, gloves, leather, etc., and the dried flowers to comfort and dry up the moisture of a cold brain.

– **Esther Singleton,** *The Shakespeare Garden,* **1922**

A tea brewed from Lavender tops, made in moderate strength, is excellent to relieve headache from fatigue and exhaustion, giving the same relief as the application of Lavender water to the temples.

– **Maude Grieve,** *A Modern Herbal,* **1931**

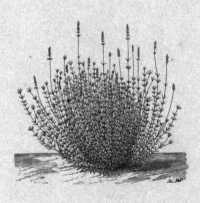

LAVENDER

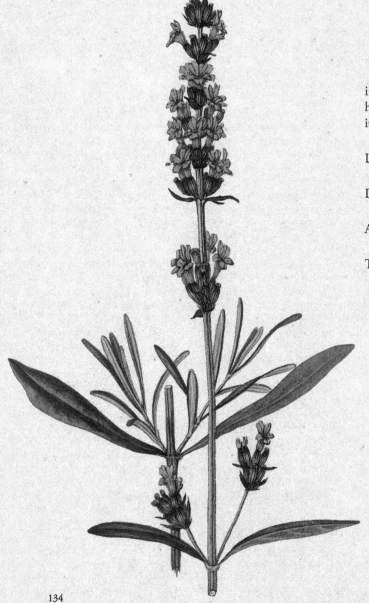

Herbal Magic

The floures of Lavender picked from the knaps, I meane the blew part and not the husk, mixed with Cinnamon, Nutmegs, & Cloves, made into powder, and given to drinke in the distilled water thereof, doth helpe the panting and passion of the heart.

– **John Gerard,** *The Herball; or, Generall Historie of Plantes,* **1636**

Because of its scent, lavender was often included in the nosegay. Lavender was much loved by sweet-hearts. In the "Handful of Pleasant Delights" (1584) it is described thus:

Lavender is for lovers true,
  Whichever more be saine,
Desiring always for to have
  Some pleasure for their pain.
And when that they have obtained have
  The love that they require,
Then have they all their perfect joy
  And quenched is the fire.

– **Esther Singleton,** *The Shakespeare Garden,* **1922**

LAVENDER

continued.

Folk Beliefs

When lavender pillows are put in a sunny apartment they are charming, and the more they are shaken up the more fragrant they become. Lavender was called by the Romans lavandula. At cutting-time people travel from long distances to inhale the fragrance of the fields. In the eighteenth century lavender-water was the principal perfume of the ladies of that period.

– *Napanee Express Newspaper,* **1910**

The expression, "laid up in lavender," is a reminder of the pleasant old custom of using the plant to scent linen. We recall Shenstone's schoolmistress whose azure lavender-spikes were bound together amidst the labour of her loom to "crown her kerchiefs clean with mickle rare perfume"; and how Keats's Madeleine slept in blanched linen, "smoothed and lavender'd." A lavender legend concerns one of the monks of the Charterhouse, a sacristan, and how he had laid the altar linen to dry in the garden. Leaving his dinner to see if all went well, he found the Virgin Mary seated beside the linen, and the Holy Child casting lavender knops thereon, as children will. So the good man said, "I may as well go to my dinner again, for the cloths are well kept." He died, they say, in 1578. An old faith was that the asp made lavender its special place of abode, and that the plant was to be approached therefore with caution.

– **Marcus Woodward,** *How to Enjoy Flowers,* **1928**

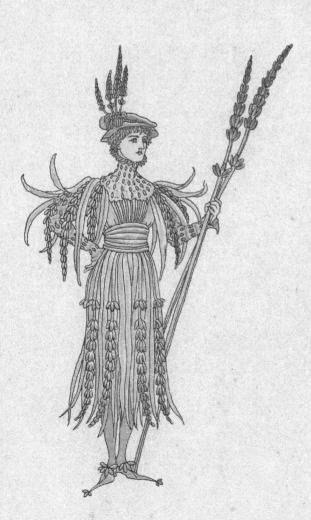

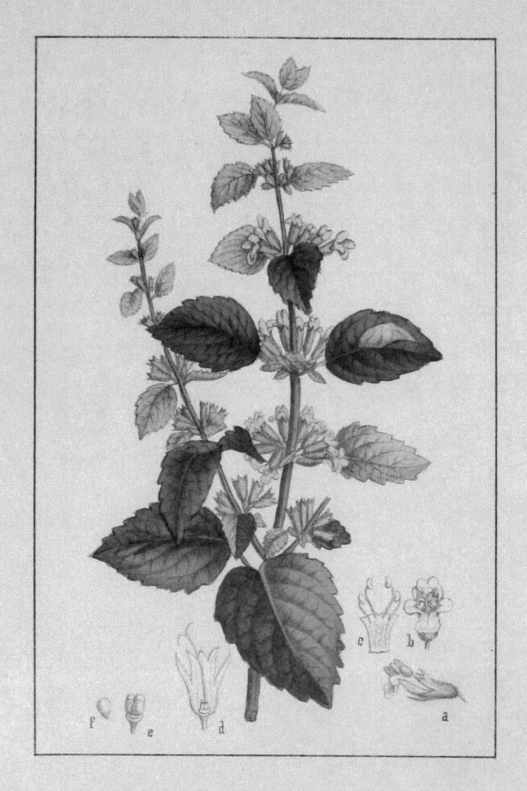

Melissa officinalis. L.

LEMON BALM

Other Names: Sweet Balm, Lemon Balsam, Melissa, Sweet Melissa
Latin Name: Melissa officinalis
Symbolises: Pleasantry
Type: Hardy herbaceous perennial
Natural Habitat: Southern Europe, in mountainous districts
Growing Zone: 3–7
Site: Tolerates light shade
Sow: March to May
Harvest: July to September
Usable Parts: Leaves
Companion Plants: Angelica, basil, borage, chamomile, echinacea,
fennel, hyssop, rosemary, sage, sweet cicely, tomatoes, and onions
Herbal Astrology: Jupiter

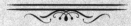

Similar in appearance to its cousins in the mint family, lemon balm's fragrant leaves are enjoyed by many for their subtle lemon flavour. It continues to hold its reputation as a calming herb, historically known for its effectiveness in soothing a restless head — believed by many to bring physical comfort and emotional cheer with its delicious aroma.

The root-stock is short, the stem square and branching, grows 1 to 2 feet high, and has at each joint pairs of broadly ovate or heart-shaped, crenate or toothed leaves which emit a fragrant lemon odour when bruised. They also have a distinct lemon taste. The flowers, white or yellowish, are in loose, small bunches from the axils of the leaves and bloom from June to October. The plant dies down in winter, but the root is perennial.

– Maude Grieve, *A Modern Herbal,* 1931

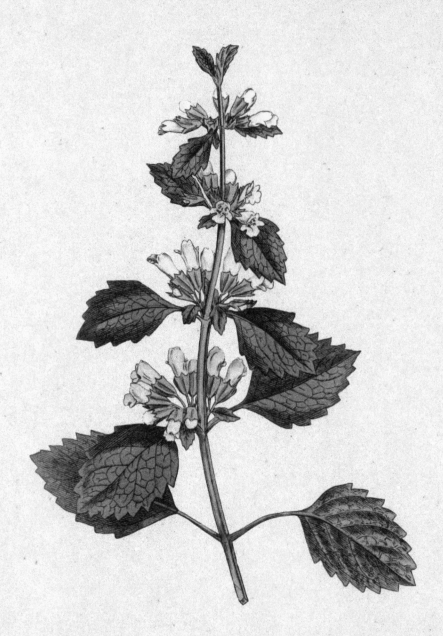

My garden grew self-heal and balm,
  And Speedwell that's blue for an hour,
Then blossoms again, O grievous my pain!
  I'm plundered of each flower.

  – 'The Sprig of Thyme', *Songs of the West*, 1928

The several chairs of order look you scour
  With juice of balm and every precious flower...

  – **William Shakespeare**, *The Merry Wives of Windsor*,
    Act 5, Scene 5, 1602

LEMON BALM continued.

In the Garden

In the herb garden a broad edging of Balm with its rich,
abundant foliage, is delightful, and it looks well with Sweet Cicely,
Angelica, and other tall-growing herbs. A low-growing edging
would be out of keeping with such herbs, but Balm in rich, moist
soil attains well over two feet, and a border of it, two feet wide,
looks very handsome. Although a native of southern Europe, Balm
has naturalized itself in the southern parts of these islands. In the
garden it is a rampant grower. It can be increased by seed, cuttings,
or division of roots in spring or autumn. It does well in any soil and
any position, but does best in full sun and moist soil.

  – Eleanour Sinclair Rohde, *Herbs and Herb Gardening,* **1936**

It is profitably planted where bees are kept. The hives of bees
being rubbed with the leaves of bawme, causeth the bees to keep
together, and causeth others to come with them.

  – John Gerard, *The Herball; or, Generall Historie of Plantes,* **1636**

It is noteworthy that in Germany the plant believed to entice
bees to the hive is also called Mutterkraut (mother herb) and is
considered healing to mothers.

  – Margaret Warner Morley, *The Honey-Makers,* **1899**

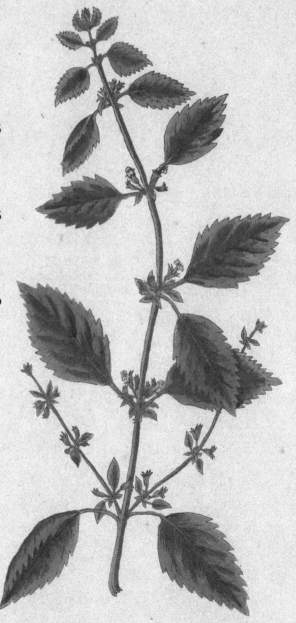

LEMON BALM

continued.

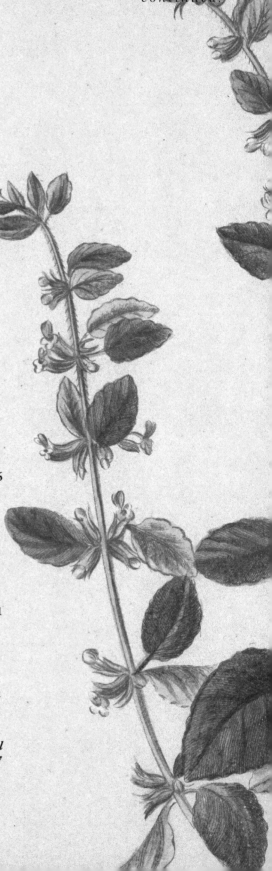

In the Kitchen

Young Balm leaves cut up finely are a good addition to mixed salads and Balm tea made by pouring boiling water on two big handfuls of the leaves has a sweet and delicate taste.

– Eleanour Sinclair Rohde, *Herbs and Herb Gardening,* **1936**

John Hussey, of Sydenham, who lived to the age of 116, breakfasted for fifty years on Balm tea sweetened with honey, and herb teas were the usual breakfasts of Llewelyn Prince of Glamorgan, who died in his 108th year. Carmelite water, of which Balm was the chief ingredient, was drunk daily by the Emperor Charles V.

– Maude Grieve, *A Modern Herbal,* **1931**

A Recipe for Carmelite Water (Compound Spirit of Balm)
Take of the fresh leaves of Balm, 8 ounces; Lemon-Peel, bruised, 4 ounces; Nutmegs and Carraway-Seeds of each, 2 ounces; Cloves, Cinnamon, Angelica Root, of each 1 ounce. Distil all together with a quart of brandy. It must then be well preserved in bottles with glass toppers.

– Nicholas Culpeper & William Joseph Simmonite, *The Herbal Remedies of Culpeper and Simmonite – Nature's Medicine,* **1957**

LEMON BALM continued.

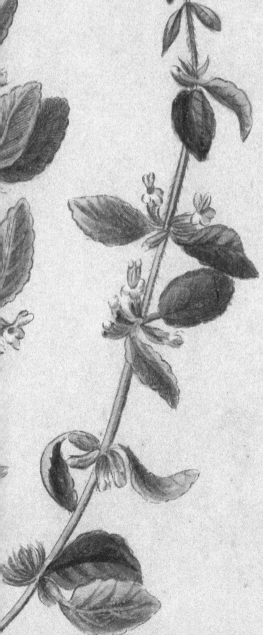

ANCIENT KNOWLEDGE, VIRTUES, AND LORE

Medicinal Properties and Remedies

It is an excellent stomachic; it braces the nerves, helps faintings, swoonings, and digestion, causes perspiration, and is therefore good in colds and headache.

— **David Ellis,** *Medicinal Herbs and Poisonous Plants*, **1918**

A Refreshing Drink in Fever:
Put a little tea-sage, two sprigs of *Balm,* and a little wood-sorrel, into a stone-jug, having first washed and dried them; peel thin a small lemon, and clear from the white; slice it and put a bit of peel in; then pour in 3 pints of boiling water, sweeten and cover it close.

— **Maria Eliza Ketelby Rundell,** *A New System of Domestic Cookery,* **1806**

Balm, like Borage, has always had the reputation of cheering the heart and dispelling sadness.

— **Eleanour Sinclair Rohde,** *Herbs and Herb Gardening,* **1936**

Homelier, yet as grateful a luxury, is the pillow of lemon balm, which displaced and derided the plant is really one of the strongest nervines, whether sipped in tea or laid under a restless head.

— **'The Woman's World',** *The Sussex Times,* **1895**

Herbal Magic

A Way to Cause Merry Dreams

When you go to bed, to eat Balm, and you cannot desire more
pleasant sights then will appear to you, fields, gardens, trees,
flowers, meadows, and all the ground a pleasant green, and covered
with shady bowers.

> — **John Baptista Porta,** *Natural Magick,* **1558**

Folk Beliefs

There is another curiously suggestive superstition connected with
this plant, which is that he who carries it with him can lead cattle
wherever he wishes.

> — **Margaret Warner Morley,** *The Honey-Makers,* **1899**

Aubrey's Legend of Balm

In the Moorlands in Staffordshire, lived a poor old man, who had
been a long time lame. One Sunday, in the afternoon, he being
alone, one knocked at his door: he bade him open it, and come in.
The Stranger desired a cup of beer; the lame man desired him to
take a dish and draw some, for he was not able to do it himself. The
Stranger asked the poor old man how long he had been ill? the poor
man told him. Said the Stranger, "I can cure you. Take two or three
balm leaves steeped in your beer for a fortnight or three weeks, and
you will be restored to your health; but constantly and zealously
serve God." The poor man did so, and became perfectly well. This
Stranger was in a purple-shag gown, such as was not seen or known
in those parts. And nobody in the street after even song did see any
one in such a coloured habit.

> — **John Aubrey,** *Miscellanies upon Various Subjects,* **1696**

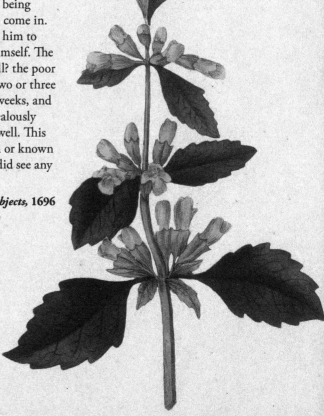

Tab. 128.

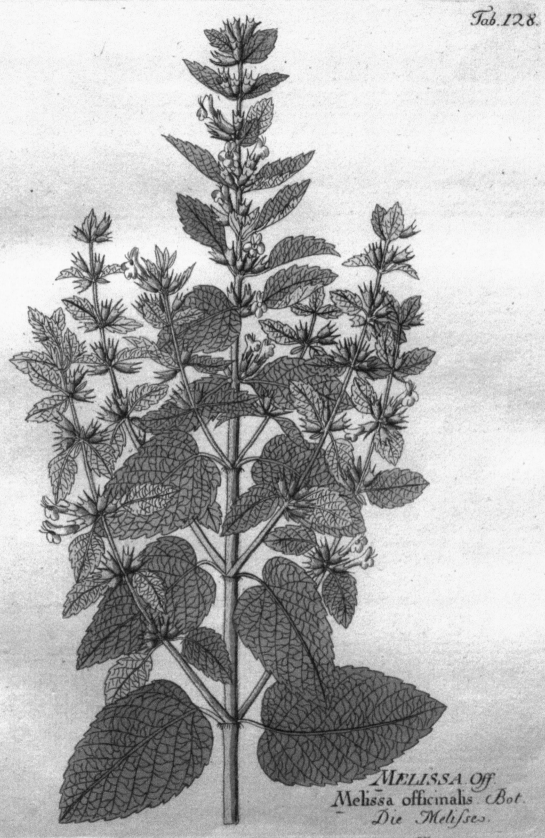

MELISSA Off.
Melissa officinalis Bot.
Die Melisse.

Tab. 116

LEVISTICUM Off.
Ligusticum Levisticum. Bot.
Das Liebstöckel

LOVAGE

Other Names: Old English Lovage, Italian Lovage, Cornish Lovage
Latin Name: Ligusticum officinale, Ligusticum levisticum
Symbolises: Abundance of desire
Type: Hardy perennial
Natural Habitat: Western Asia, parts of the Middle East,
and the Mediterranean region
Growing Zone: 4
Site: Sun or partial shade
Sow: Autumn or spring
Harvest: June to August
Usable Parts: Stem, leaves, root, and seeds
Companion Plants: Catmint, fennel, and hyssop
Herbal Astrology: The Sun

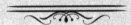

Entirely edible, lovage boasts a crisp citrussy taste similar to celery or parsley. Its leaves make a lovely addition to summer salads, while its seeds can be used to flavour soups and stocks. It was once believed that a potent remedy could be created from the seeds, supposed to have the ability to restore dull eyesight. It is a joy to have in the herb garden and is easy to grow and maintain.

It has many long and green stalks of large winged leaves, divided into many parts, like Smallage, but much larger and greater, every leaf being cut about the edges, broadest forward, and smallest at the stalk, of a sad green colour, smooth and shining; from among which rise up sundry strong, hollow green stalks, five or six, sometimes seven or eight feet high, full of joints, but lesser leaves set on them than grow below; and with them towards the tops come forth large branches, bearing at their tops large umbels of yellow flowers, and after them flat brownish seed. The roots grow thick, great and deep, spreading much, and enduring long, of a brownish colour on the outside, and whitish within. The whole plant and every part of it smelling strong, and aromatically, and is of a hot, sharp, biting taste.

– Nicholas Culpeper, *Complete Herbal,* **1824**

LOVAGE

continued.

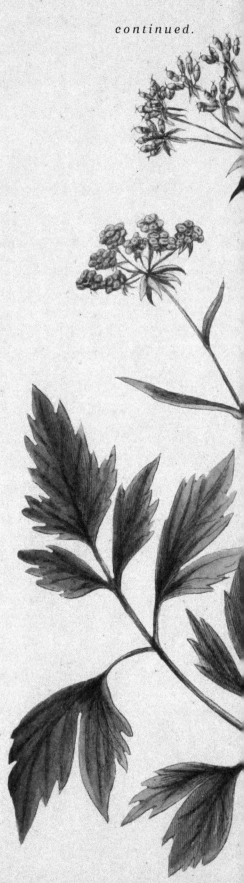

In the Garden

Lovage requires a deep, rich, moist soil, and should be sown in August, or immediately after ripening. When the young plants have grown three inches, transplant them three feet apart in each direction. When they are well established they will require but little care and will continue for years.

– Jules Arthur Harder, *The Physiology of Taste*, 1885

In the Kitchen

The root has a strongly aromatic fragrance, the leaves have an aromatic, fruit-like scent with a suggestion of Parsley scent, the stalks smell rather like Celery and the seeds are very aromatic. We always include a leaf of Lovage finely chopped in our salads for the taste is most pleasant and unusual.

– Eleanour Sinclair Rohde, *Herbs and Herb Gardening*, 1936

Both the roots and seeds are used. The roots are sliced and dried and are used by confectioners in that state.

– Jules Arthur Harder, *The Physiology of Taste*, 1885

Candied Lovage

Cut the young stems in April and boil in water till tender, then drain very carefully. Scrape slightly and dry carefully in a cloth, and lay in a syrup previously prepared. Leave three days with the vessel well covered, then heat but do not let the syrup boil. When it is thoroughly heated lay the pieces on a dish to dry—near the fire.

– Hilda Leyel, *Herbal Delights*, 1937

LOVAGE *continued.*

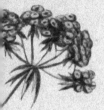

ANCIENT KNOWLEDGE, VIRTUES, AND LORE

Medicinal Properties and Remedies

Lovage was much used as a drug plant in the fourteenth century, its medicinal reputation probably being greatly founded on its pleasing aromatic odour.

The roots and fruit are aromatic and stimulant, and have diuretic and carminative action. In herbal medicine they are used in disorders of the stomach and feverish attacks, especially for cases of colic and flatulence in children, its qualities being similar to those of Angelica in expelling flatulence, exciting perspiration and opening obstructions. The leaves eaten as salad, or infused dry as a tea, used to be accounted a good emmenagogue.

An infusion of the root was recommended by old writers for gravel, jaundice and urinary troubles, and the cordial, sudorific nature of the roots and seeds caused their use to be extolled in 'pestilential disorders.'

– Maude Grieve, *A Modern Herbal,* **1931**

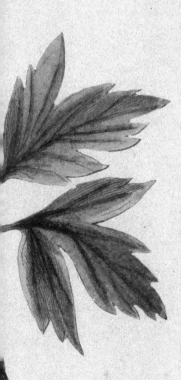

It is a known and much praised remedy to drink the decoction of the herb for any sort of ague, and to help the pains and torments of the body and bowels coming of cold. The seed is effectual to all the purposes aforesaid (except the last) and works more powerfully. The distilled water of the herb helps the quinsy in the throat, if the mouth and throat be gargled and washed therewith, and helps the pleurisy, being drank three or four times. Being dropped into the eyes, it takes away the redness or dimness of them.

Remedy:
Half a dram at a time of the dried root in powder taken in wine, doth wonderfully warm a cold stomach, helps digestion.

– Nicholas Culpeper, *Complete Herbal,* **1824**

For ache in the Knees.
Take Rue and Lovage, of each alike, stamp them, and mix them with Honey, and fry them together, and lay a Plaister thereof warm to the sore.

– Bahia, *The Skilful Physician,* **1656**

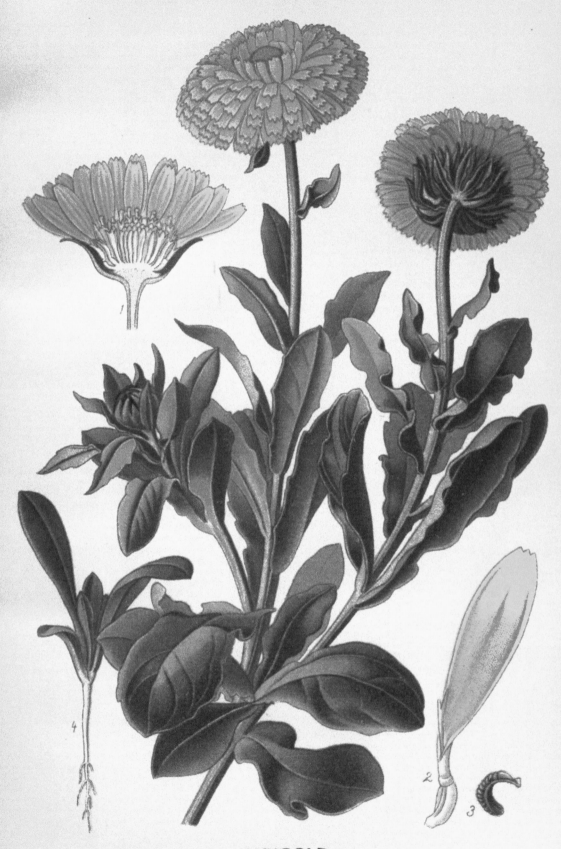

MARIGOLD

(CALENDULA OFFICINALIS)

Nat. size

PL. 155

MARIGOLD

Other Names: Calendula, Golds, Mary Gooles, Ruddes
Latin Name: Calendula officinalis
Symbolises: Grief
Type: Half-Hardy Annual
Natural Habitat: Southern Europe, the Levant
Growing Zone: 2–11
Site: Full sun
Sow: March to May
Harvest: When in full bloom
Usable Parts: Flowers, leaves, and whole herb
Companion Plants: Comfrey, horehound, and savory
Herbal Astrology: The Sun

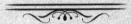

A small yet bright flower, marigolds have been common in gardens for centuries. The yellow flowers have been traditionally associated with the sun due to their bright appearance, with their vivid heads said to follow the sun's path in the sky throughout the day. They were often dried and steeped in water or wine to create a soothing tisane to calm the head and heart. Nowadays, they make a charming ingredient in summer salads, adding a pop of colour and mellow flavour.

The Marigold has enjoyed great and lasting popularity, and though the flower does not charm by its loveliness, the indomitable courage, with which, after even a sharp frost, it lifts up its hanging head, and shows a cheerful countenance, leads one to feel for it affection and respect.

– **Rosalind Northcote,** *The Book of Herbs,* **1903**

They are the richest yellow of all garden flowers, and no modern introductions can compare with the vivid splendour of their golden colouring. Great drifts of Marigolds in sunlight are almost dazzling.

– **Eleanour Sinclair Rohde,** *Herbs and Herb Gardening,* **1936**

MARIGOLD

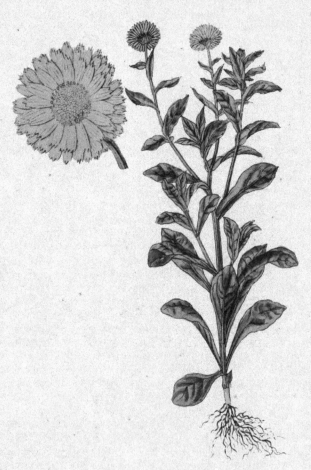

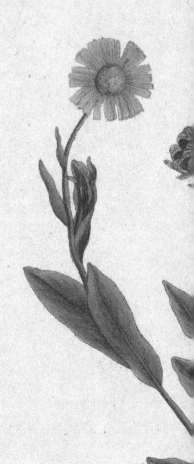

Open afresh your round of starry folds,
Ye ardent marigolds!
Dry up the moisture from your golden lids,
For great Apollo bids
That in these days your praises should be sung

– John Keats, 'I stood tiptoe upon a little hill', 1816

The Marigold observes the sun,
More than my subjects me have done.

– King Charles I

...So shuts the marigold her leaves
At the departure of the sun;
So from the honeysuckle sheaves
The bee goes when the day is done...

– William Browne, 'Memory', 1613

...The marigold, that goes to bed wi' the sun,
And with him rises weeping:...

**– William Shakespeare, *A Winter's Tale*,
Act 4, Scene 4, 1623**

MARIGOLD continued.

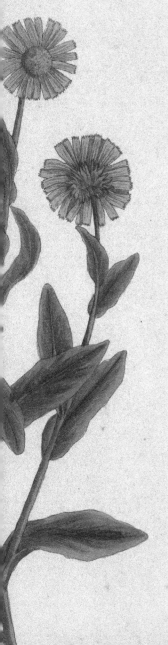

In the Garden

The Marigold floureth from Aprill or May even untill Winter, and in Winter also, if it bee warme. It is called Calendula: it is to be seene in floure in the Calends almost of every moneth.

— **John Gerard**, *The Herball; or, Generall Historie of Plantes*, **1636**

In order to keep plants grown from seed in pots or pans short and sturdy, they should be pricked off into other pots as soon as big enough to handle, after this they may be hardened off ready for planting out in late May or early June.

— **John William Morton**, *250 Beautiful Flowers and How to Grow Them*, **1939**

The instructions for the picking of this joyous flower are given at length. It must be taken only when the moon is in the sign of the Virgin, and not when Jupiter is in the ascendant, for then the herb loses its virtue.

— **Eleanour Sinclair Rohde**, *The Old English Herbals*, **1922**

In the Kitchen

The dried petals were used in broths and stews, and Gerard states that the demand for them was so great that in the grocers' shops they were stored in barrels. "No broths," he concludes, "are well made without dried Marigolds." The flowers were also used to impart a yellow colour to cheese. Marigold puddings were made with the petals finely chopped, cream, and breadcrumbs mixed and baked. The flowers were also used in pickles and cordials, and Charles Carter, who was Cook to the Duke of Argyll in 1737, gives a recipe for Marigold wine in his Recipe Book. The petals are still not infrequently used salads by those who do not object to eating flowers. The young leaves are also edible, but seldom used.

— **Eleanour Sinclair Rohde**, *Herbs and Herb Gardening*, **1936**

MARIGOLD WINE. Boil three pounds and a half of lump sugar in a gallon of water, put in a gallon of marigold flowers, gathered dry and picked from the stalks, and then make it as for cowslip wine. If the flowers be gathered only a few at a time, measure them when they are picked, and turn and dry them in the shade. When a sufficient quantity is prepared, put them into a barrel, and pour the sugar and water upon them. Put a little brandy into the bottles, when the wine is drawn off.

— **Mary Eaton**, *The Cook and Housekeeper's Complete and Universal Dictionary*, **1822**

151

MARIGOLD

continued.

ANCIENT KNOWLEDGE, VIRTUES, AND LORE

Medicinal Properties and Remedies

It has been cultivated in the kitchen garden for the flowers, which are dried for broth, and said to comfort the heart and spirits.

– Maude Grieve, *A Modern Herbal*, 1931

The flowers of Marigold were much used by American surgeons during the Civil War, in treating wounds, and with admirable results. "Calendula owes its introduction and first use altogether to homoeopathic practice, as signally valuable for healing wounds, ulcers, burns, and other breaches of the skin surface." Personal experience leads me to suggest that it is an excellent household remedy.

– Rosalind Northcote, *The Book of Herbs*, 1903

A tea made of the fresh flowers gathered of the Marigold, picked from the cups, is good in fevers; it gently promotes perspiration, and throws out anything that ought to appear on the skin.

– Nicholas Culpeper & William Joseph Simmonite, *Herbal Remedies of Culpeper and Simmonite*, 1957

An infusion of marigold-flowers is given to patients suffering from scarlet fever, measles, and eruptions of the skin. A couple of handfuls of the flowers are boiled in a quart of water, and a wineglassful given to the sufferer, who must be kept warm.

– Isabella Beeton, *Gardening*, 1861

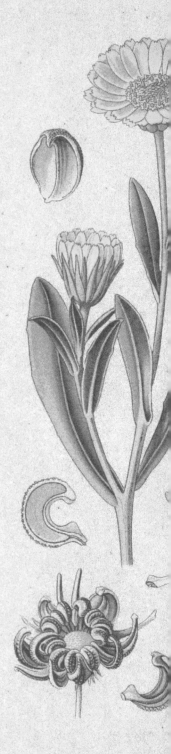

MARIGOLD

continued.

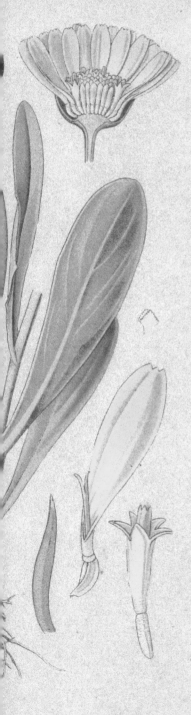

Herbal Magic

"If thou hast a mind to see in thy dream the man thou wilt marry, follow my direction and you shall not fail. . . . Take marigold flowers and a sprig of marjoram and thyme. Dry them before the fire in a piece of white muslin, and when they are dry, rub them to powder. With this mix a little vinegar and honey till all is a paste. On going to bed anoint your lips with this paste, and afterwards say aloud:

> *Lover's friend, be kind to me,*
> *Let me now my true love see.*

"Then hasten to sleep and in your night's repose the man you are to marry will appear beside your bed, walking to and fro, very plain to be seen. You shall perfectly behold his visage, stature and deportment, and if he be one that will prove a loving husband, he will be seen to smile. But if the marriage is to prove unhappy you will see him frowning and uncivil."

— **Diana Hawthorne,** *Laurie's Complete Fortune Teller,* **1946**

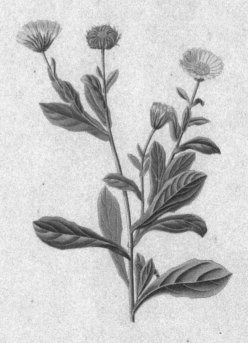

MARIGOLD *continued.*

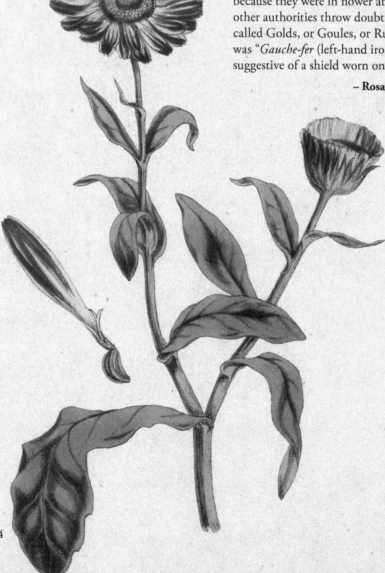

Folk Beliefs

The Latin name refers to its reputed habit of blossoming on the first days of every month in the year, and in a fairly mild winter this is no exaggeration. Marigolds are dedicated to the Virgin, but this fact is not supposed to have had anything to do with the giving of their name, which had probably been bestowed on them before the Festivals in her honour were kept in England, "Though doubtless," says Mr. Friend, "the name of Mary had much to do with the alterations in the name of marigold, which may be noticed in its history." There is an idea that they were appropriated to her because they were in flower at all of her Festivals; but on this notion other authorities throw doubt. In ancient days marigolds were often called Golds, or Goules, or Ruddes; in Provence, a name for them was "*Gauche-fer* (left-hand iron) probably from its brilliant disc, suggestive of a shield worn on the left arm."

– Rosalind Northcote, *The Book of Herbs,* **1903**

MARIGOLD

continued.

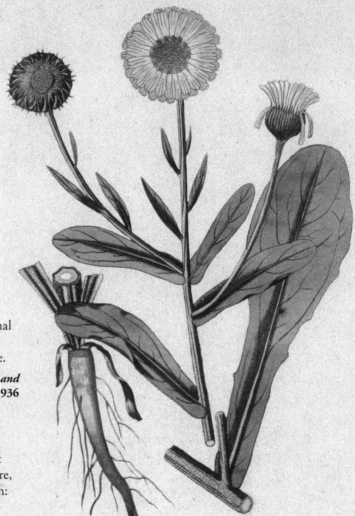

Joseph Hall, who was Bishop of Exeter in the first half of the seventeenth century, wrote a beautiful passage about Marigolds in his Occasional Meditations, comparing the faithful soul to the Marigold ever turning to the Sun and Lord of Life.

– **Eleanour Sinclair Rohde,** *Herbs and Herb Gardening,* 1936

On the Sight of Marigolds

These flowers are true clients of the sun: how observant they are of his motion and influence! At even, they shut up; as mourning from his departure, without whom they neither can nor would flourish: in the morning, they welcome his rising, with cheerful openness: and at noon, are fully displayed, in a free acknowledgment of his bounty.

Thus doth the good heart unto God. *When though turned away thy face, I was troubled;* saith the man after God's own heart. Thus doth the carnal heart to the world: when that withdraws his favour, he is dejected; and revives, with a smile. All is in our choice. Whatsoever is our sun will thus carry us.

O God, be though to me, such as thou art in thyself: thou shalt be merciful, in drawing me; I shall be happy, in following thee.

– **Joseph Hall,** *The Works of Joseph Hall,* 1808

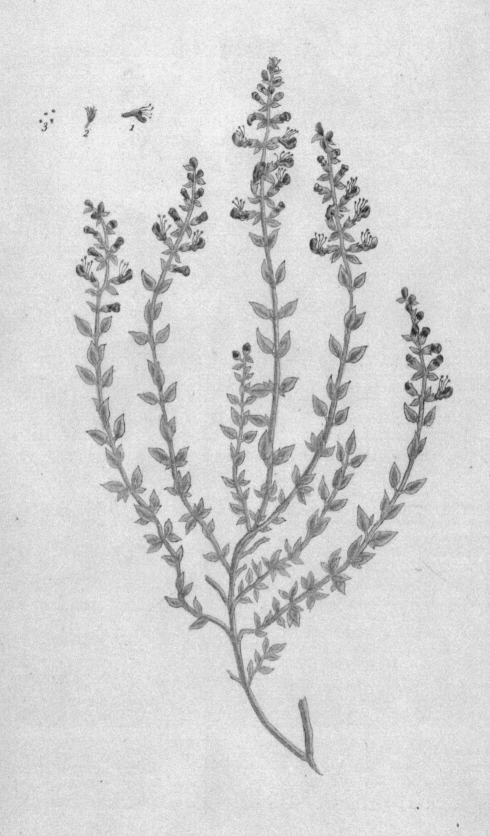

Marum

1 Flower
2 Cup
3 Seed

Marum feryacum

MARJORAM

Other Names: Knotted Marjoram, Sweet Marjoram
Latin Name: Origanum majorana
Symbolises: Blushes and joy
Type: Herbaceous Perennial
Natural Habitat: Asia, North Africa, Europe, including Great Britain
Growing Zone: 9–10
Site: Sunny, sheltered spot
Sow: February to May
Harvest: June to October
Usable Parts: Leaves and stem
Companion Plants: Basil, chives, oregano, parsley, rosemary, sage, thyme, and lavender
Herbal Astrology: Mercury

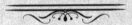

Delicate and sensitive to the cold, marjoram is a beautiful herb. It has a long history as a medicinal herb, most commonly known now as a digestive aid. Its pine and citrus flavours lend themselves to savoury and sweet dishes – working well with sauces, soups, and stews. To make marjoram tea, steep dried leaves in hot water and add honey for extra sweetness.

The quiet charm and warm aromatic scents of the Marjorams appeal to all those who love old-fashioned flowers (…) Like most wildlings, isolated clumps of wild Marjoram look out of place in a border, but in the herb garden this plant looks at home. It makes a delightful edging and broad borders of its pleasant, deliciously scented flowers are homely and pleasant. In Tudor and Stuart times Marjoram and Thrift were apparently the only herbaceous plants used for making Knots, for which purpose the dwarf shrubs were more commonly used. Thomas Hyll, in his *Proffitable Arte of Gardening* gives a plan of a knot to be set with "Marjoram and such like, or Isope and Time"

– Eleanour Sinclair Rohde, *Herbs and Herb Gardening*, 1936

MARJORAM

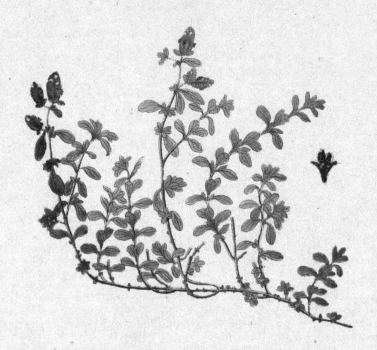

With marjoram knots, sweet-brier, and ribbon-grass,
And lavender, the choice of ev'ry lass,
And sprigs of lad's love – all familiar names,
Which every garden through the village claims.

– John Clare, 'June', 1827

My soul is like a garden-close
  Where marjoram and lilac grow,
  Where soft the scent of long ago
Over the border lightly blows.

Where sometimes homing winds at play
  Bear the faint fragrance of a rose –
  My soul is like a garden close
Because you chanced to pass my way.

– Thomas S. Jones, Jr., 'My Soul Is Like a Garden-Close', 1911

MARJORAM

continued.

In the Garden

The Marjorams are fond of a dry situation, and this is no exception to that rule. Rockwork or raised beds of sandy loam suits it to perfection, provided the aspect is sunny. It will, therefore, be seen that there is nothing special about its culture, neither is there in its propagation; cuttings may be taken in summer, or the rooted shoots may be divided at almost any time. It flowers from September to the time of severe frosts, and is in its greatest beauty in October.

– John Wood, *Hardy Perennials and Old-Fashioned Garden Flowers,* **1884**

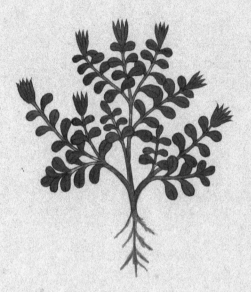

Sow the seeds as early as possible and thin out the plants to ten inches apart. It is also propagated by dividing the roots either in spring or autumn.

– Jules Arthur Harder, *The Physiology of Taste,* **1885**

In the Kitchen

Few people know how to keep the flavor of sweet-marjoram; the best of all herbs for broth and stuffing. It should be gathered in bud or blossom, and dried in a tin-kitchen at a moderate distance from the fire; when dry, it should be immediately rubbed, sifted, and corked up in a bottle carefully.

– Lydia Maria Child, *The American Frugal Housewife,* **1829**

This herb gives a delicious flavour to soups, sauces and seasonings; and is nice (dried and powdered) sprinkled over roast pork just before serving.

– Florence White, *Good Things in England,* **1932**

MARJORAM

continued.

ANCIENT KNOWLEDGE, VIRTUES, AND LORE

Medicinal Properties and Remedies

Marjoram possesses stimulant and carminative properties. It is also regarded as a mild tonic and diaphoretic; and was formerly held in great repute as an emmenagogue. It may be used for similar purposes as the mints... the dried leaves have been used as a substitute for China tea.

> – **Robert Bentley**, *Medicinal Plants*, 1880

A strong infusion makes an excellent hair restorer. When the hair is weak and falling, a nightly massage with this infusion will work wonders.

> – **Mary Thorne Quelch**, *A Guide to your Herb Garden*, 1951

In common with the majority of the old herbalists, Gerard had a faith in herbs which was simple and unquestioning. Sweet marjoram, he tells us, is for those "who are given to over-much sighing."

> – **Eleanour Sinclair Rohde**, *The Old English Herbals*, 1922

And the dry leaves made into powder, mixed with Honey, and anointed upon any part, doth take away black and blew spots of the skin. The Oyl made thereof is very warming, and comfortable to the joynts which are stiff.

[It] is a chief Ingredient in most of those Powders that Barbers use, in whose Shops I have seen great store of this Herb hanged up.

> – **William Coles**, *Adam in Eden; Or, Natures Paradise, The History of Plants*, 1657

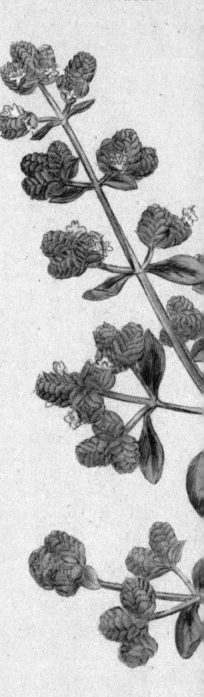

MARJORAM _continued._

Herbal Magic

German mothers placed horehound or snapdragon (Orant is the German name), black cumin, blue marjoram, a right shirt-sleeve and a black, left stocking. Then the fairies (Nickerts in German) could not injure the child.

– M. A. Radford & E. Radford, *Encyclopaedia of Superstitions – A History of Superstition,* **1947**

Folk Beliefs

When Venus carried off the sleeping Ascanius to the groves of Idalia, she laid him amidst Marjoram. Virgil probably referred to Sweet Knotted Marjoram (Origanum majorana). Few herbs have been so esteemed for scent and for culinary purposes through the centuries. For its scent it was valued as a strewing herb and as such Tusser lists it in his Five Hundred Points (1577). Gerard described the scent as "marvelous sweet" and "aromaticall", and amongst other uses he prescribed a decoction of the leaves "for such as are given to over-much sighing". In his Countrie Housewife's Garden (1618) Lawson divided the garden into two parts, the one to contain "the hearbes and flowers used to make nosegaies and garlands" and the other "all other sweet-smelling hearbes", and of this garden, in which he places Marjoram, he says: "And this may be called the Garden for hearbes of a good smell."

According to Parkinson, Sweet Marjoram was used "to please the outward senses in nosegays and in the windows of houses, as also in sweete powders, sweet bags, and sweete washing waters".

– Eleanour Sinclair Rohde, *Herbs and Herb Gardening,* **1936**

Plate 12.

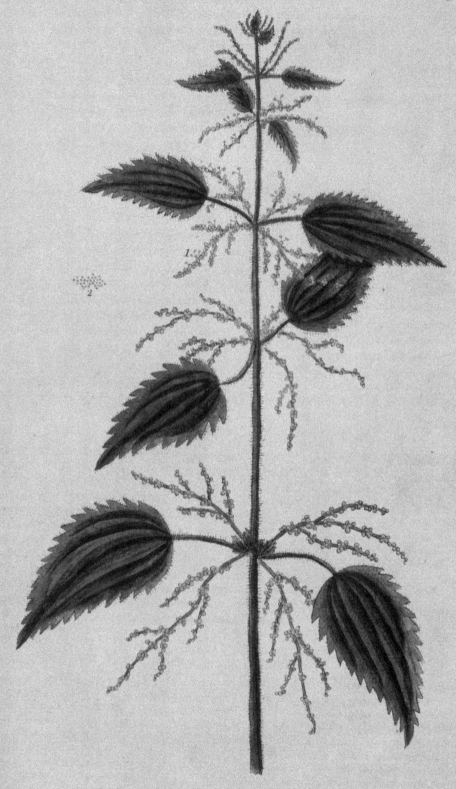

Eliz. Blackwell delin. sculp. et Pinx.

Stinging Nettle

{ 1 *Flower* {
{ 2 *Seed* {

Urtica

NETTLE

Other Names: Stinging Nettle, Common Nettle, Burn Nettle, Stinger
Latin Name: Urtica dioica
Symbolises: Spitefulness, burning – slander
Type: Herbaceous perennial
Natural Habitat: Europe, including Great Britain; Africa, Australia
Growing Zone: 4–10
Site: Full sun to partial shade, in moist soil
Sow: October to December
Harvest: March to April
Usable Parts: Herb and seeds
Companion Plants: Chard, kale, and spinach
Herbal Astrology: Mars

More often than not, nettles are seen as common weeds, found nestled among hedgerows and growing uninhibited in gardens everywhere. While they are most well known for their stinging properties, they are a diverse and nutritious ingredient in the kitchen. Delicious when cooked into soups and purees, the leaves and flowers can be used for all sorts of recipes – even dried and steeped in tea. Soaking or cooking the nettles will remove the stingers so they can be eaten without injury. To avoid being stung when harvesting, make sure to wear gloves.

Nettles are so well known, that they need no description; they may be found by feeling, in the darkest night.

– Nicholas Culpeper, *Complete Herbal,* **1824**

The Nettle tribe, Urticaceae, is widely spread over the world and contains about 500 species, mainly tropical, though several, like our common Stinging Nettle, occur widely in temperate climates. Many of the species have stinging hairs on their stems and leaves. Two genera are represented in the British Isles, Urtica, the Stinging Nettles, and Parietaria, the Pellitory (…) The British species of Stinging Nettle, belonging to the genus Urtica (the name derived from the Latin, uro, to burn), are well known for the burning properties of the fluid contained in the stinging hairs with which the leaves are so well armed.

– Maude Grieve, *A Modern Herbal,* **1931**

NETTLE

continued.

TENDER-HANDED stroke a nettle,
　And it stings you for your pains;
Grasp it like a lad of mettle,
　And it soft as silk remains.
'Tis the same with grov'ling natures;
　Use them kindly they rebel:
But be rough as nutmeg graters,
　And the rogues obey you well.

**– Aaron Hill (1685-1750), 'Verses Written on a
Window in Scotland'**

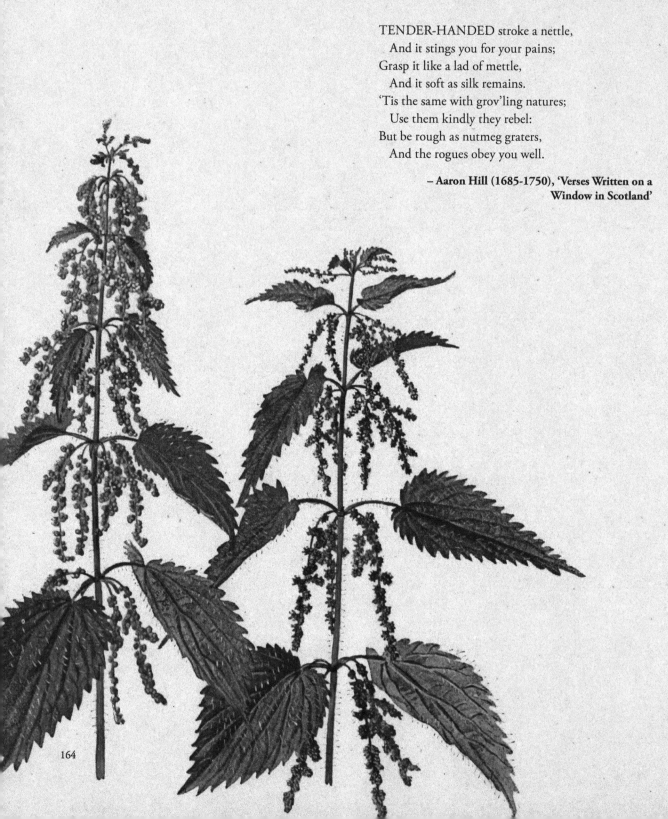

164

NETTLE

continued.

In the Garden

Early in April the tops will furnish tender leaves that are used as a pot herb for soups, or are prepared the same as spinach. The cultivated Nettle is used most, being propagated from roots that are planted either in pots or in the forcing house. They will soon send up an abundance of tender tops. They may be blanched by covering them with other pots. If planted close to a flue in the vineyard they will produce excellent Nettle-kale or Nettle-spinach in January or February.

– Jules Arthur Harder, *The Physiology of Taste,* **1885**

In the Kitchen

From a culinary point of view the Nettle has an old reputation. It is one of the few wild plants still gathered each spring by country-folk as a pot-herb. It makes a healthy vegetable, easy of digestion.

– Maude Grieve, *A Modern Herbal,* **1931**

To make nettle (or sorrel) soup. Wash and boil as for spinach, and rub the leaves through a sieve. Melt a little butter in a stewpan and sprinkle in an ounce of flour, add the mashed nettles, and (a little at a time) sufficient milk to make a soup of the required thickness—it should not be too thick; bring to the boil, simmer for 5 minutes, season with pepper and salt, and serve with diced croutons of fried bread. A pair of scissors and gardening gloves are useful when gathering nettles.

– L. C. R. Cameron, *The Wild Foods of Great Britain,* **1917**

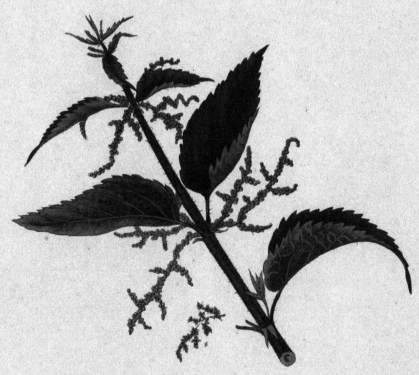

NETTLE

continued.

ANCIENT KNOWLEDGE, VIRTUES, AND LORE

Medicinal Properties and Remedies

This is also an herb Mars claims dominion over. You know Mars is hot and dry, and you know as well that Winter is cold and moist; then you may know as well the reason why Nettle-tops eaten in the Spring consume the phlegmatic superfluities in the body of man, that the coldness and moistness of Winter hath left behind. The roots or leaves boiled, or the juice of either of them, or both made into an electuary with honey and sugar, is a safe and sure medicine to open the pipes and passages of the lungs, which is the cause of wheezing and shortness of breath, and helps to expectorate tough phlegm, as also to raise the imposthumed pleurisy; and spend it by spitting; the same helps the swelling of the almonds of the throat, the mouth and throat being gargled therewith. The juice is also effectual to settle the palate of the mouth in its place, and to heal and temper the inflammations and soreness of the mouth and throat.

— **Nicholas Culpeper,** *Complete Herbal,* **1824**

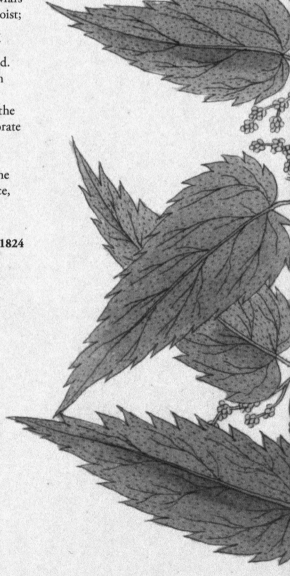

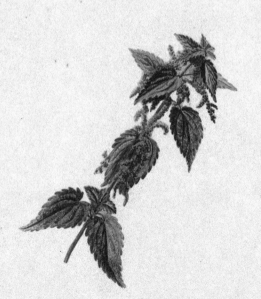

NETTLE

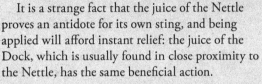

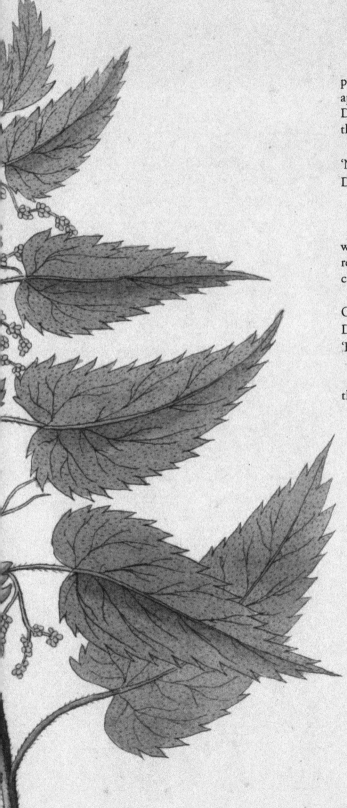

It is a strange fact that the juice of the Nettle proves an antidote for its own sting, and being applied will afford instant relief: the juice of the Dock, which is usually found in close proximity to the Nettle, has the same beneficial action.

'Nettle in, dock out.
Dock rub nettle out!'

is an old rhyme.

If a person is stung with a Nettle a certain cure will be effected by rubbing Dock leaves over the part, repeating the above charm slowly. Another version is current in Wiltshire:

Out 'ettle in dock,
Dock zhail ha' a new smock;
'Ettle zhant ha' narrun! (none)

The sting of a Nettle may also be cured by rubbing the part with Rosemary, Mint or Sage leaves.

– Maude Grieve, *A Modern Herbal*, 1931

NETTLE

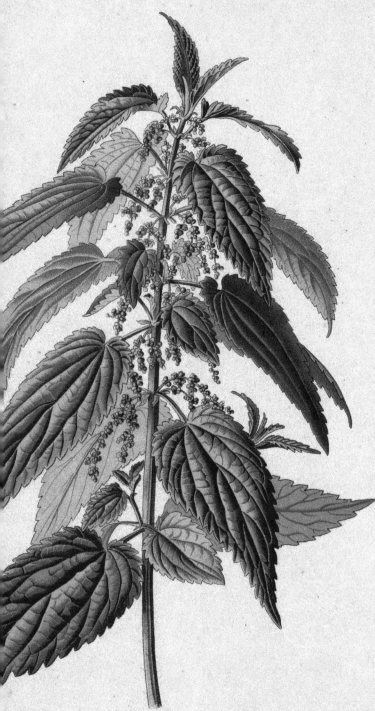

A decoction of the nettle, often known as St. Fabian's nettle, is a favourable prescription among countrywomen for consumption; and in Scotland there is a story related of a mermaid of the Firth of Clyde who, on seeing the funeral of a young girl who had died of consumption, exclaimed:—

"If they wad drink nettles in March,
   And eat muggins* in May,
Sae mony braw maidens
   Wadna gang to the clay."

– Robert Chambers, *Popular Rhymes of Scotland,* **1826**
*Mugwort

The seed being drank, is a remedy against the stinging of venomous creatures, the biting of mad dogs, the poisonous qualities of Hemlock, Henbane, Nightshade, Mandrake, or other such like herbs that stupify or dull the senses; as also the lethargy, especially to use it outwardly, to rub the forehead or temples in the lethargy, and the places stung or bitten with beasts, with a little salt.

An ointment made of the juice, oil, and a little wax, is singularly good to rub cold and benumbed members. An handful of the leaves of green Nettles, and another of Wallwort, or Deanwort, bruised and applied simply themselves to the gout, sciatica, or joint aches in any part, hath been found to be an admirable help thereunto.

– Nicholas Culpeper, *Complete Herbal,* **1824**

NETTLE

Herbal Magic

To dream you see nettles is a warning of trouble. To dream you are stung by nettles is a sign you have difficulty. To dream you see other people stung by nettles is a sign of unexpected news.

– **Diana Hawthorne,** *Laurie's Complete Fortune Teller,* **1946**

As evil is an antidote for evil, the nettle held in the hand is a guard against ghosts, and it is good for beer when laid upon the barrel.

– **Charles Godfrey Leland,** *Gypsy Sorcery and Fortune Telling,* **1891**

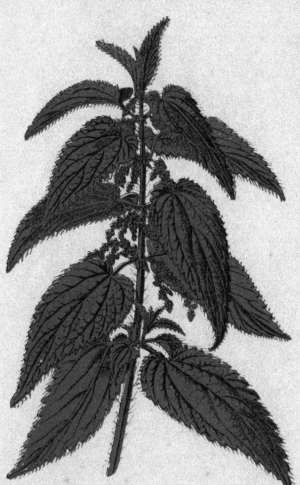

Folk Beliefs

It is, or was, occasionally stewed into a tea by country women and administered to the helpless and unfortunate as a cure for anything that might be the matter with them. It is one of the five bitter herbs which the Jews were commanded to eat at the Passover. The Roman nettle, that thrives in England, was planted there by Cæsar's soldiers, who, not having breeches thick enough to enable them to withstand the climate, suffered much in the cold, raw fogs; so, when their legs were numb they plucked nettles and gave those members such a scouring that they burned and smarted gloriously for the rest of the day.

– **Charles Montgomery Skinner,** *Myths and Legends of Flowers, Trees, Fruits and Plants,* **1911**

The seed of it, according to Nicander, is an antidote to the poison of hemlock of fungi, and of quicksilver. Apollodorus prescribes it, too, taken in the broth of a boiled tortoise, for the bite of the salamander, and as an antidote for the poison of henbane, serpents, and scorpions.

– **Elder Pliny,** *The Natural History of Pliny,* **c. 77 AD**

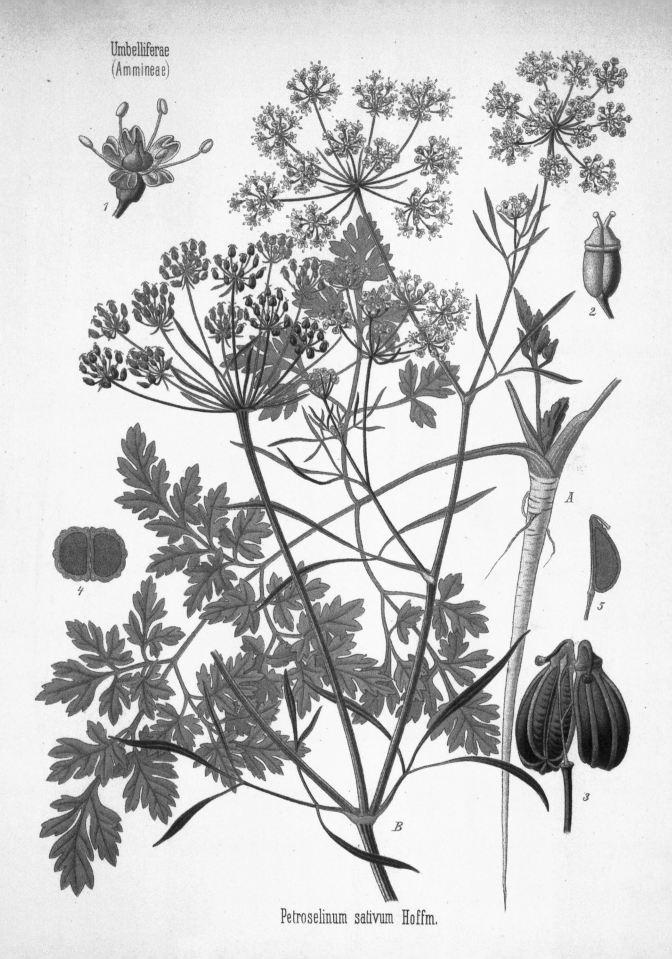

Petroselinum sativum Hoffm.

PARSLEY

Other Names: Scent Leaf, Garden Parsley
Latin Name: Petroselinum crispum
Symbolises: Joy and festivity
Type: Annual
Natural Habitat: Sardinia
Growing Zone: 4–9
Site: Full sun or partial shade
Sow: March to May
Harvest: Three months after planting
Usable Parts: Leaves, stem, and seeds
Companion Plants: Basil, chives, dill, fennel, lavender, lemon balm, marjoram,
oregano, rosemary, sage, savory, and thyme
Herbal Astrology: Mercury

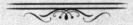

*A versatile culinary herb, parsley's peppery taste is used in recipes worldwide. It
prospers well in the garden nearby dill and coriander, offering abundant green foliage
throughout the summer while hardy enough to sustain well into the autumn months.
Pick the leaves regularly to encourage new growth.*

The Garden Parsley is not indigenous to Britain: Linnaeus stated its wild
habitat to be Sardinia, whence it was brought to England and apparently
first cultivated here in 1548. Bentham considered it a native of the Eastern
Mediterranean regions; De Candolle of Turkey, Algeria and the Lebanon. Since
its introduction into these islands in the sixteenth century it has been completely
naturalized in various parts of England and Scotland, on old walls and rocks.

– Maude Grieve, *A Modern Herbal,* **1931**

PARSLEY

continued.

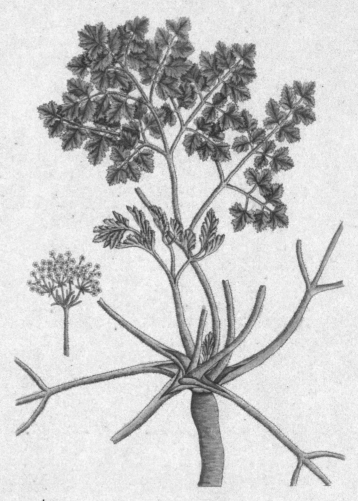

And where the marjoram once, and sage, and rue,
And balm, and mint, with curl'd-leaf parsley grew,
And double marygolds, and silver thyme,
And pumpkins 'neath the window us'd to climb;
And where I often when a child for hours
Tried through the pales to get the tempting flowers,
As lady's laces, everlasting peas,
True-love-lies-bleeding, with the hearts-at-ease,
And golden rods, and tansy running high,
That o'er the pale-tops smil'd on passers-by.

– John Clare, 'The Cross Roads; or, The Haymaker's Story', 1821

PARSLEY

continued.

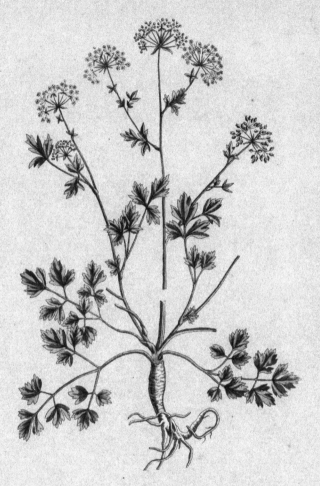

In the Garden

Parsley is a biennial, though generally grown as an annual, because the leaves from young plants are much the best; the seeds should be sown two or three times a year, beginning about February, in a sheltered nook; this herb likes plenty of sun; even the curliest varieties degenerate if placed in a damp shady situation. It prefers light soil, and gives a better winter supply than where the soil is heavy. Flower-heads must be cut off regularly to keep the plants in good condition, though just a few of the best kinds may be allowed to perfect their seed, which should be sown as soon as ripe.

– Violet Biddle, *Small Gardens and How to Make the Most of Them,* 1901

Parsley to be used for drying has always to be sown early. For summer use the April sowing is the most useful. Plants to stand the winter are sown in August. Early thinning is essential to secure first-rate Parsley. In spells of drought the rows need liberal watering. As a rule the plants are of little or no value after their second year.

– Eleanour Sinclair Rodhe, *Herbs and Herb Gardening,* 1936

The seed lies a long time in the ground before it germinates, from thirty-five to forty days. It is generally planted as an edging, or border; but if a bed is wanted it should be sown in drills eight inches apart. It bears seed the second year, and then dies away; but to preserve the border when the tendency of the stalks to run displays itself, they should be cut off. The seed dropping in the ground, however, will renew the border from time to time of itself, though it will upon these occasions wear a "scraggy" appearance.

– Isabella Beeton, *Gardening,* 1861

In the Kitchen

The uses of Parsley are many and are by no means restricted to the culinary sphere. The most familiar employment of the leaves in their fresh state is, of course, finely-chopped, as a flavouring to sauces, soups, stuffings, rissoles, minces, etc., and also sprinkled over vegetables or salads. The leaves are extensively cultivated, not only for sending to market fresh, but also for the purpose of being dried and powdered as a culinary flavouring in winter, when only a limited supply of fresh Parsley is obtainable.

In addition to the leaves, the stems are also dried and powdered, both as a culinary colouring and for dyeing purposes.

— **Maude Grieve,** *A Modern Herbal,* **1931**

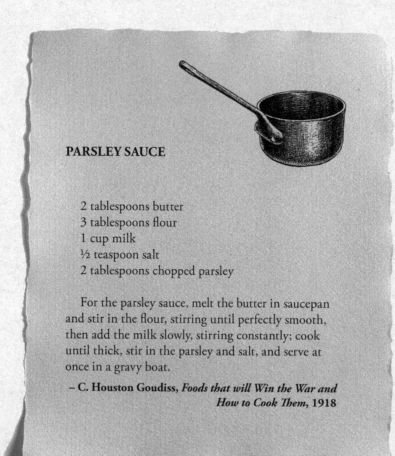

PARSLEY SAUCE

2 tablespoons butter
3 tablespoons flour
1 cup milk
½ teaspoon salt
2 tablespoons chopped parsley

For the parsley sauce, melt the butter in saucepan and stir in the flour, stirring until perfectly smooth, then add the milk slowly, stirring constantly; cook until thick, stir in the parsley and salt, and serve at once in a gravy boat.

— **C. Houston Goudiss,** *Foods that will Win the War and How to Cook Them,* **1918**

Parsley is mostly in request as a garnish, or for putting into melted butter; for the latter purpose, it must be well washed and chopped fine and put into the sauce just before it is sent to table.

Fried Parsley.—After having been picked and washed, the parsley must be shaken in a cloth until thoroughly dry, then turned into a pan of boiling hot fat; it should be fried quickly, and taken out the moment it is crisp, put in a coarse cloth to drain, or on a sheet of paper in a Dutch oven before the fire, and turned quickly until quite crisp.

— **Tom Jerrold,** *Our War-Time Kitchen Garden: The Plants We Grow and How We Cook Them,* **1917**

PARSLEY

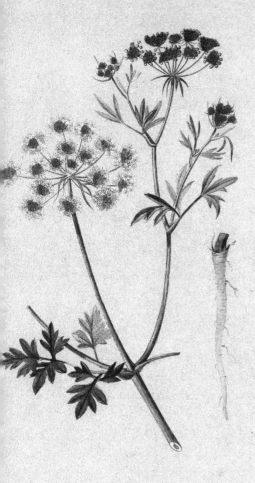

ANCIENT KNOWLEDGE, VIRTUES, AND LORE

Medicinal Properties and Remedies

COMMON Garden Parsley is under Mercury, and strengthens the stomach, is diuretic, or provokes urine, menses, wind in the bowels; it is an aperient.

For falling sickness, jaundice, dropsy, stone, pain in the kidneys, take Parsley, Fennel, Anise, and Carraway Seeds, 1 ounce; Roots of Parsley, Burnet, Saxifrage, and Carraways, 1/2 ounce. Boil in 2 pints of water down to 1, then strain; and take a cupful two or three times a day.

– Nicholas Culpeper & William Joseph Simmonite, *Herbal Remedies of Culpeper and Simmonite,* 1957

For all evills within the Bladder.
Take Fennell seeds, Parsley seeds, and Smalladge seeds; bruise them and temper them with faire running Water, and drink this first and last at your pleasure.

– Ralph Williams, *A Black Almanack or Predictions and Astronimonicall Observations,* 1651

Herbal Magic

So they say that fumes made with linseed, flea-bane seed, roots of violets, and parsley, doth make one to foresee things to come and doth conduce to prophesying.

– Henry Cornelius Agrippa, *The Philosophy of Natural Magic,* 1913

Parsley thrown into fish ponds will heal the sick fishes therein.

– Eleanour Sinclair Rohde, *The Old English Herbals,* 1922

PARSLEY

continued.

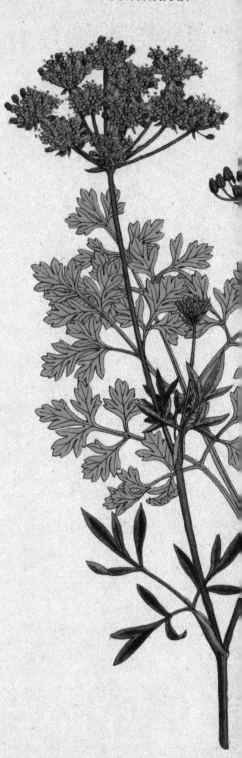

Folk Beliefs

There is an old superstition against transplanting parsley plants. The herb is said to have been dedicated to Persephone and to funeral rites by the Greeks. It was afterwards consecrated to St. Peter in his character of successor to Charon.

The Greeks held Parsley in high esteem, crowning the victors with chaplets of Parsley at the Isthmian games, and making with it wreaths for adorning the tombs of their dead. The herb was never brought to table of old, being held sacred to oblivion and to the dead. It was reputed to have sprung from the blood of a Greek hero, Archemorus, the forerunner of death, and Homer relates that chariot horses were fed by warriors with the leaves. Greek gardens were often bordered with Parsley and Rue.

– **Maude Grieve,** *A Modern Herbal,* **1931**

Parsley was used, too, to strew on graves, and hence came a saying, "to be in need of parsley", signifying to be at death's door.

(…)

It is one of the longest seeds to lie in the ground before germinating; it has been said to go to the Devil and back again nine times before it comes up. Any many people have a great objection to planting parsley, saying if you do there will sure to be a death in the family within twelve months.

– **Rosalind Northcote,** *The Book of Herbs,* **1903**

PARSLEY

continued.

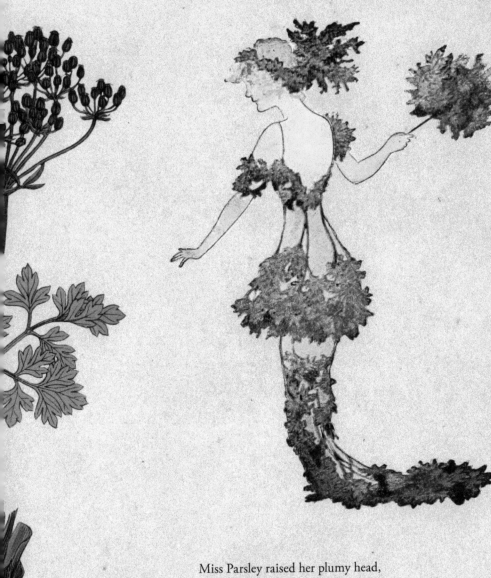

Miss Parsley raised her plumy head,
And in her modest manner said:
"I'm only asked to dine, I know,
Because my dress becomes me so!"

– Elizabeth Gordon, *Mother Earth's Children,* **1914**

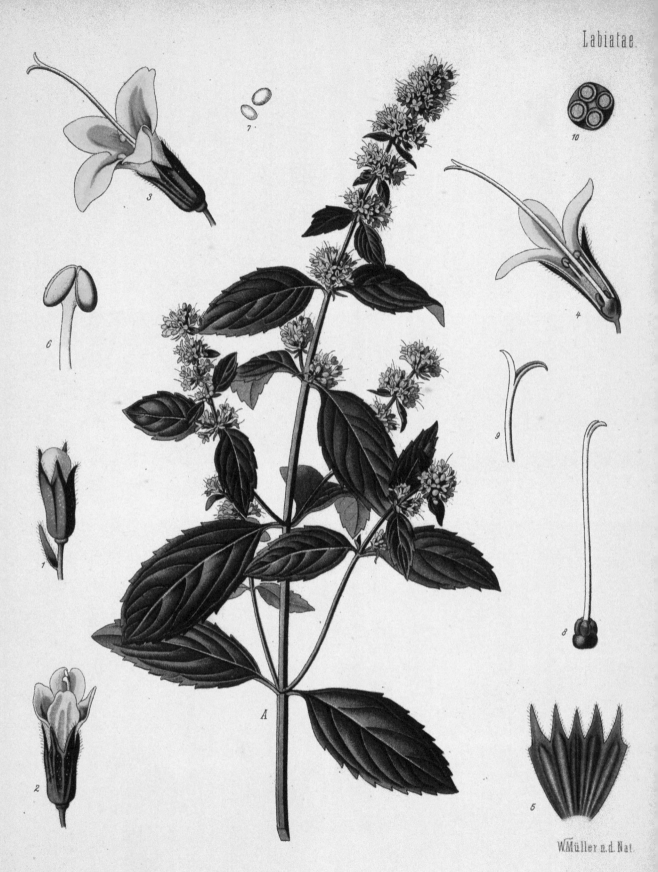

Labiatae.

Mentha piperita L.

WMüller n.d. Nat.

PEPPERMINT

Other Names: Brandy Mint, Lily-Rail
Latin Name: Mentha piperita
Symbolises: Warmth of feeling
Type: Perennial herb
Natural Habitat: Europe and Asia
Growing Zone: 5–10
Site: Partial shade or full sun
Sow: February to June or August to September
Harvest: Regularly once established
Usable Parts: Leaves and stem
Companion Plants: Brassicas, oregano, peas, and tomatoes
Herbal Astrology: Venus

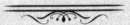

A popular choice from the mint family, peppermint is a classic and cherished addition to the herb garden. A hybrid species of watermint and spearmint, it is a fierce and abundant grower and is best to plant in pots to keep it contained. A delicious tea can be made by steeping fresh leaves in hot water – the perfect digestive after a meal.

The plant is found throughout Europe, in moist situations, along stream banks and in waste lands, and is not infrequent in damp places in England, but is not a common native plant, and probably is often an escape from cultivation. In America it is probably even more common as an escape than Spearmint, having long been known and grown in gardens.

Of the members of the mint family under cultivation the most important are the several varieties of the Peppermint (Mentha piperita), extensively cultivated for years as the source of the well-known volatile oil of Peppermint, used as a flavouring and therapeutic agent.

– Maude Grieve, *A Modern Herbal,* **1931**

PEPPERMINT

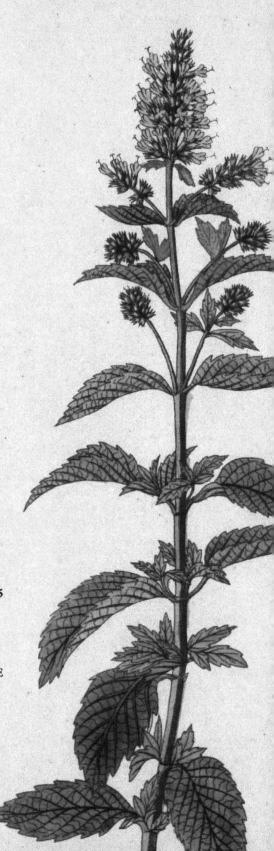

What small leaf-fingers veined with emerald light
Lay on my heart that touch of elfin might?

What spirals of sharp perfume do they fling,
To blur my page with swift remembering?

Borne in a country basket marketward,
Their message is a music spirit-heard,

A pebble-hindered lilt and gurgle and run
Of tawny singing water in the sun.

Their coolness brings that ecstasy I knew
Down by the mint-fringed brook that wandered through

My mellow meadows set with linden-trees
Loud with the summer jargon of the bees.

Their magic has its way with me until
I see the storm's dark wing shadow the hill

As once I saw: and draw sharp breath again,
To feel their arrowy fragrance pierce the rain.

O sudden urging sweetness in the air,
Exhaled, diffused about me everywhere,

Yours is the subtlest word the summer saith,
And vanished summers sigh upon your breath.

– Grace Walcott Hazard Conkling, 'A Breath of Mint', 1915

"Then rubb'd it o'er with newly-gather'd Mint,
A wholesom Herb, that breath'd a grateful Scent."

– Ovid, 'The Metamorphoses', Book 8, c. 8 CE

PEPPERMINT

continued.

In the Garden

This plant is propagated either by parting the roots, or by slipped roots of the young spring plants being taken up with plenty of root fibres; also by cuttings during April, May, etc. But at this season the best and most universal method used is to part the roots.

Any time this month have recourse to such old beds of mint as are well stocked with young plants. Cut and draw up enough of the strongest shoots properly rooted. Draw them up gently, with the help of your knife, to raise or separate them. Every plant will rise with tolerably good roots.

Plant in rows about six inches apart, and five or six inches distant in the rows; also well water, to settle the soil closely about the roots.

To propagate mint by roots, get a quantity of old roots, part them, then draw drills with a hoe six inches apart; place the roots in the drills, cover them about an inch deep with the earth, and then rake the ground.

The roots should be procured and planted either in February or the beginning of this month (March), or in October or November.

The plants will thrive in almost any soil or situation. They will quickly take root and grow very freely, producing a crop the same year, and these roots will produce a crop annually for many years.

– **C. D. McKay,** *The French Garden,* **1908**

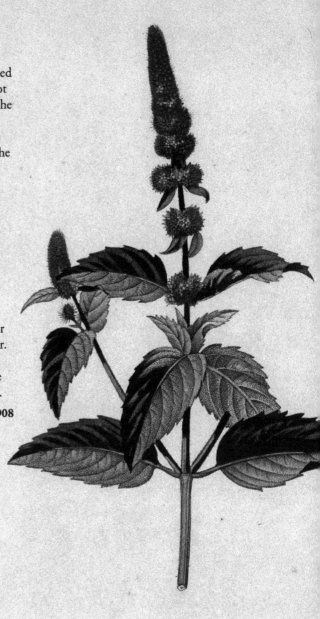

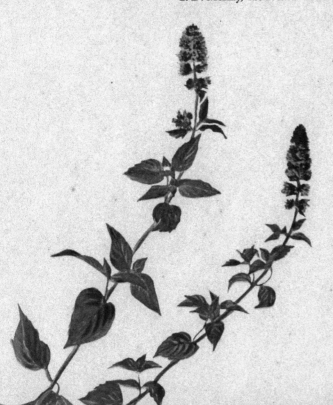

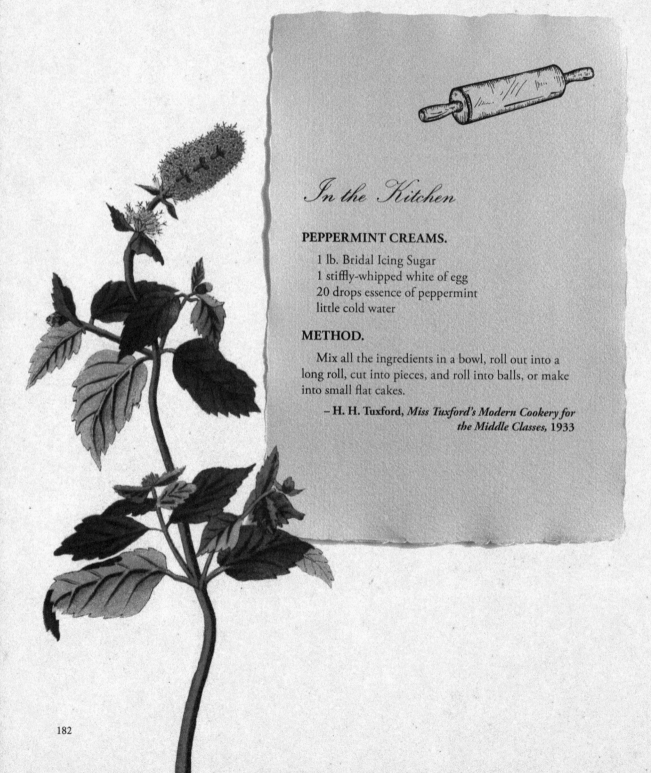

In the Kitchen

PEPPERMINT CREAMS.

1 lb. Bridal Icing Sugar
1 stiffly-whipped white of egg
20 drops essence of peppermint
little cold water

METHOD.

Mix all the ingredients in a bowl, roll out into a long roll, cut into pieces, and roll into balls, or make into small flat cakes.

– H. H. Tuxford, *Miss Tuxford's Modern Cookery for the Middle Classes*, 1933

PEPPERMINT

continued.

ANCIENT KNOWLEDGE, VIRTUES, AND LORE

Medicinal Properties and Remedies

It is good for wind and colic in the stomach, to procure the menses, and expel the birth and secundines. The juice dropped into the ears eases the pains of them. The juice laid on warm, helps scrofula, or kernels in the throat. The decoction or distilled water helps a stinking breath, proceeding from corruption of the teeth; and snuffed up the nose, purges the head. It helps the scurf or dandruff of the head used with vinegar.

— Nicholas Culpeper & William Joseph Simmonite, *The Herbal Remedies of Culpeper and Simmonite,* 1957

In slight colds or early indications of disease, a free use of Peppermint tea will, in most cases, effect a cure, an infusion of 1 ounce of the dried herb to a pint of boiling water being employed, taken in wineglassful doses; sugar and milk may be added if desired.

— Maude Grieve, *A Modern Herbal,* 1931

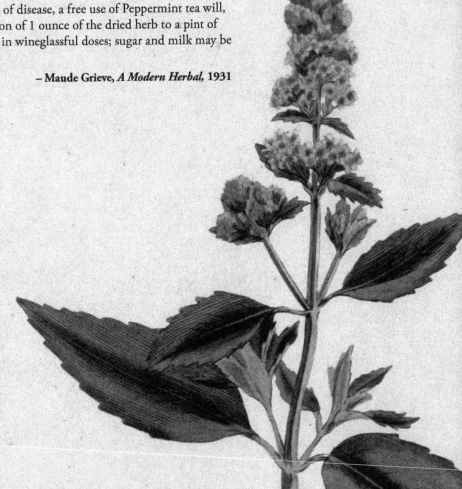

PEPPERMINT

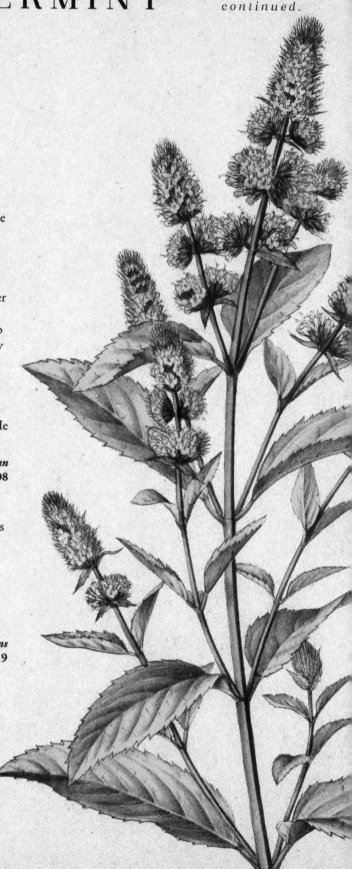

continued.

Herbal Magic

Sarah Smith, the wife of a marine store dealer, residing at Golden Hill, was for some time ill and confined to her bed. Finding that the local doctor could not cure her, she sent for a witch doctor of Taunton. He duly arrived by train on St. Thomas's day. Smith inquired his charge, and was informed he usually charged 11s., remarking that unless he took it from the person affected his incantation would be of no avail. Smith then handed it to his wife, who gave it to the witch doctor, and he returned 1s. to her. He then proceeded to foil the witch's power over his patient by tapping her several times on the palm of her hand with his finger, telling her that every tap was a stab on the witch's heart. This was followed by an incantation. He then gave her a parcel of herbs (which evidently consisted of dried bay leaves and peppermint), which she was to steep and drink. She was to send to a blacksmith's shop and get a donkey's shoe made, and nail it on her front door. He then departed.

— **George Laurence Gomme,** *Folklore as an Historical Science,* **1908**

A Charm to Cause Love

Keep a sprig of mint in your hand till the herb grows moist and warm, then take hold of the hand of the woman you love, and she will follow you as long as the two hands close over the herb. No invocation is necessary; but silence must be kept between the two parties for ten minutes, to give the charm time to work with due efficacy.

— **Jane Wilde,** *Mystic Charms and Superstitions of Ireland,* **1919**

PEPPERMINT

continued.

Folk Beliefs

Mint of every kind was held in high esteem by the Romans, and in telling the story of Baucis and Philemon, the poor old couple whom the gods visited disguised as weary travellers, Ovid describes how the hosts scoured the table with mint to lend it a pleasant scent in honour of the guests, whose identity they did not discover until the visit was ending.

The ancients served mint in milk, believing that the herb would prevent the milk from curdling. In comparatively recent times the idea was dismissed as an idle superstition and yet the older farmers hereabouts insist that if the cows eat generously of wild mint their milk is useless for cheese-making, and old wives say that a poultice of freshly gathered mint leaves should be applied hot to a woman's breasts for resolving the coagulated milk.

Bees are attracted to mint flowers and bee-keepers tell you there is no danger of a new hive being deserted if it has been well rubbed with freshly gathered mint leaves before the introduction of the bees to their new home.

> – **Mary Thorne Quelch**, *A Guide to Your Herb Garden*, 1951

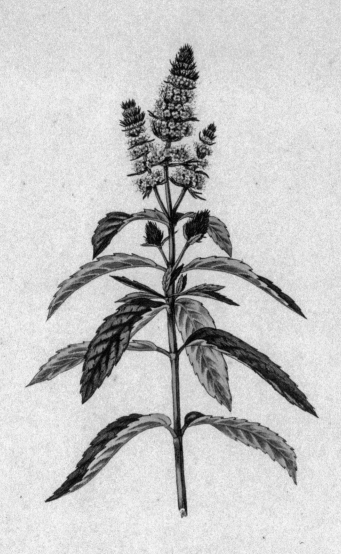

Plate 159.

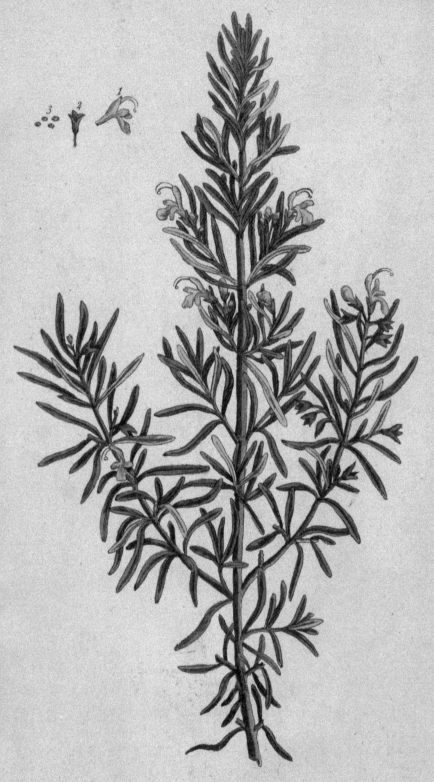

Rosemary.

Eliz. Blackwell delin. sculp. et Pinx.

1. Flower separate.
2. Calix.
3. Seed.

Rosmarinus.

ROSEMARY

Other Names: Dew of the Sea, Polar plant, Compass plant
Latin Name: Rosmarinus officinalis
Symbolises: Remembrance
Type: Evergreen shrub
Natural Habitat: Southern and central Europe
Growing Zone: 8–9
Site: Sunny, sheltered spot
Sow: March to April
Harvest: All year
Usable Parts: Leaves and flowers
Companion Plants: Bay, basil, chives, fennel, lavender, lemon verbena, marjoram, oregano, parsley, sage, savory, tarragon, and thyme
Herbal Astrology: The Sun

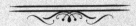

As delightful planted alone or in boundaries and borders, legend states that rosemary will only grow well when tended to by women. If planted on the edges of pathways, its fragrant stems release their scent when brushed past, making it the perfect addition to those seeking a scented garden. The new growth in the early summer is the most flavoursome for those wishing to cook with it, either used fresh or dried for later use.

Rosemary—"dew of the sea"—is poetically and aptly named. Not only is the colouring of the plant with the rich green of the upper surfaces of the leaves and the grey undersides suggestive of the sea, but its delicious smell has something of the tang of sea salt in it. Possibly the name is due to the picturesque appearance of the shrub when the new shoots have grown. The old leaves stand out almost horizontally, but on the new shoots they are stiffly upright, thereby affording a contrast between the grey undersides displayed and the rich green of the older leaves, showing their upper sides, on the lower growths of the bush. The contrast is certainly suggestive of the dark green and grey of a troubled sea.

– Eleanour Sinclair Rodhe, *Herbs and Herb Gardening*, 1936

ROSEMARY

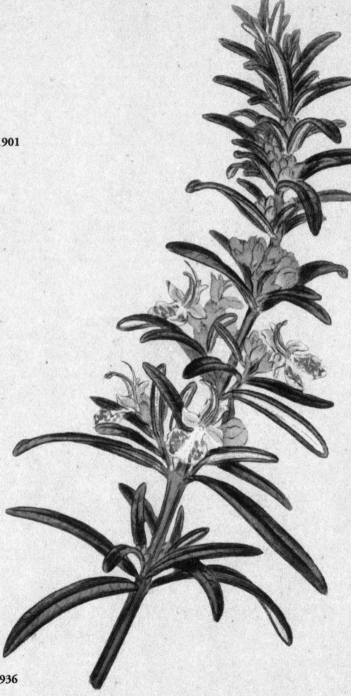

Sweet herbs in plenty, blue borage
And the delicious mint and sage,
Rosemary, marjoram, and rue,
And thyme to scent the winter through.

     – Kartharine Tynan, 'The Choice', 1901

    THERE once was a lady, divinely tall,
     Who lived high up in a castle wall,
     And longed to be lord in her husband's hall.

A troubadour chanced to be passing by,
As the lady looked down from her casement high.

He stood at the foot of the castle wall,
And sang to the lady, divinely tall,
Who longed to be lord in her husband's hall:

"A holy father, from over the sea,
Has brought me this cutting of Rosemary.

"Plant it carefully by the wall.
If it grows a tree, both healthy and tall,
You shall be lord in your husband's hall."

The lady listened, and so it befell.
She wore the doublet and hose as well.

And even to-day
There are cynics who say:
The wife who means to master her man
Will trot down the path with her watering-can—

And if you follow her, you will see
She always waters her Rosemary.

     – Reginald Arkell, 'Legend of Rosemary', 1936

ROSEMARY

continued.

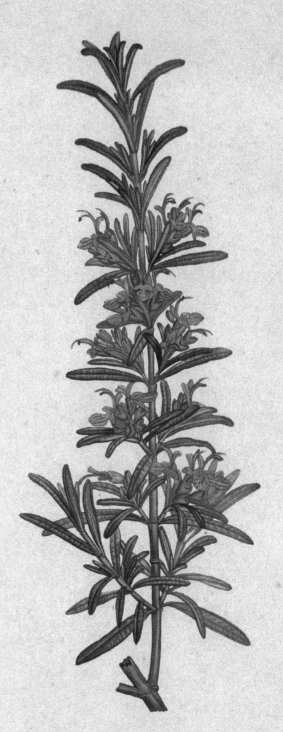

Here's Rosemary for you, that's for remembrance
> — William Shakespeare, *Hamlet*, Act 4, Scene 5, 1603

In the Garden

The Rosemary in deep free soils attains a height of 6 to 8 feet, and should find a place in every shrubbery or mixed flower-garden. It flowers in winter or early spring, and flourishes on the coast.
> — J. W. Bean, *Hardy Ornamental Trees and Shrubs*, 1897

Requires no regular pruning, but towards the end of April cut off long ends of shoots to shape the bush and clip hedges of Rosemary. Trim long shoots again in early August.
> — H. H. Thomas, *Pruning Made Easy – How to Prune Rose Trees, Fruit Trees and Ornamental Trees and Shrubs*, 1927

In the Kitchen

Rosemary is known to most people and used by very few. It can be added to stews, salads and summer drinks.
> — Various, *Gleanings from Gloucester Housewives*, 1936

Conserve of Rosemary
Pick the flowering heads when dry, rub them off the stem and sift them through a sieve, then weigh them and to every pound add 2 1/2 pounds of loaf sugar. Beat together in a stone mortar, adding the sugar by degrees. When thoroughly incorporated, press into jars without first boiling. Cover well, putting leather over the paper covers and it will keep seven years.
> — Hilda Leyel, *Herbal Delights*, 1937

ANCIENT KNOWLEDGE, VIRTUES, AND LORE

Medicinal Properties and Remedies

The young tops, leaves and flowers can be made into an infusion, called Rosemary Tea, which, taken warm, is a good remedy for removing headache, colic, colds and nervous diseases, care being taken to prevent the escape of steam during its preparation. It will relieve nervous depression. A conserve, made by beating up the freshly gathered tops with three times their weight of sugar, is said to have the same effect.

– **Maude Grieve,** *The Modern Herbal,* **1931**

Rosemary has been known for generations as providing an oil of particular value to the hair. The stimulating properties of the oil are present in the Extract, which forms an admirable dressing for the hair, especially for those with a tendency to premature greyness.

– **King Press,** *The Famous Book of Herbs,* **2013**

Hair Stimulant
Rosemary (Rosemarinus officinalis).
Boil one ounce in a pint of water for five minutes. Rub the liquid well into the scalp at night.

– **Gipsy Petulengro,** *Romany Remedies and Recipes,* **1935**

If a garland thereof be put about the head, it comforteth the brain, the memorie, the inward senses and comforteth the heart and maketh it merry.

– **John Gerard,** *The Herball; or, Generall Historie of Plantes,* **1636**

Herbal Magic

If a maid is curious as to her future, she may obtain information by dipping a spray of rosemary into a mixture of wine, rum, gin, vinegar, and water in a vessel of ground glass. She is to observe this rite on the eve of St, Magdalen, in an upper room, in company with two other maids, and each must be less than twenty-one years old. Having fastened the sprigs in their bosoms and taken three sips of the tonic — sips are quite enough — all three go to rest in the same bed without speaking. The dreams that follow will be prophetic.

– **Charles Montgomery Skinner,** *Myths and Legends of Flowers, Trees, Fruits and Plants,* **1911**

ROSEMARY

Of Rosemary in Banckes's Herbal:

- Take the flowers thereof and make powder thereof and binde it to thy right arme in a linnen cloath and it shale make thee light and merrie.

- Take the flowers and put them in thy chest among thy clothes or among thy Bookes and Mothes shall not destroy them.

- Boyle the leaves in white wine and washe thy face therewith and thy browes and thou shalt have a faire face.

- Also put the leaves under thy bedde and thou shalt be delivered of all evill dreames.

- Take the leaves and put them into wine and it shall keep the wine from all sourness and evill savours and if thou wilt sell thy wine thou shalt have goode speede.

- Also if thou be feeble boyle the leaves in cleane water and washe thyself and thou shalt wax shiny.

- Also if thou have lost appetite of eating boyle well these leaves in cleane water and when the water is colde put thereunto as much of white wine and then make sops, eat them thereof wel and thou shalt restore thy appetite againe.

- If thy legges be blowen with gowte boyle the leaves in water and binde them in a linnen cloath and winde it about thy legges and it shall do thee much good.

- If thou have a cough drink the water of the leaves boyld in white wine and ye shall be whole.

- Take the Timber thereof and burn it to coales and make powder thereof and rubbe thy teeth thereof and it shall keep thy teeth from all evils. Smell it oft and it shall keep thee youngly.

- Also if a man have lost his smellyng of the ayre that he may not draw his breath make a fire of the wood and bake his bread therewith, eate it and it shall keepe him well.

- Make thee a box of the wood of rosemary and smell to it and it shall preserve thy youth.

— **Eleanour Sinclair Rohde**, *The Old English Herbals,* 1922

ROSEMARY

continued.

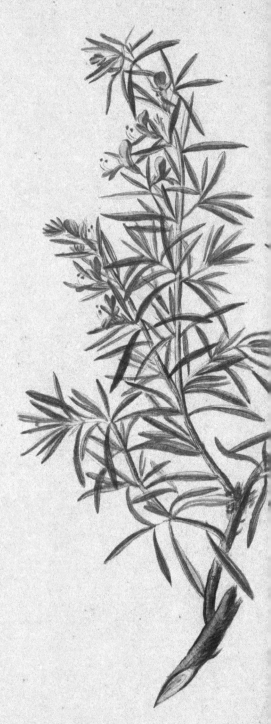

Folk Beliefs

There is a vulgar belief in Gloucestershire and other counties, that Rosemary will not grow well unless where the mistress is "master"; and so touchy are some of the lords of creation upon this point, that we have more than once had reason to suspect them of privately injuring a growing rosemary in order to destroy this evidence of their want of authority.

— **Maude Grieve,** *The Modern Herbal,* **1931**

Would you know the secret of eternal youth, my good woman? It is to sleep on a rosemary pillow. I like the rosemary best when it is in flower.

— **Marcus Woodward,** *The Mistress of Stantons Farm,* **1938**

This plant, which is not a rose and is not dedicated to Mary, takes its name from the Latin, rosmarinum, or sea dew, for it is fond of the water. The Romans made decorative as well as ceremonial use of rosemary, crowning with it the guests at banquets, employing it in funeral rites, wreathing it on their household gods, and purifying their flocks with its smoke. They believed that the odor of the plant tended to preserve the bodies of the dead, and the lasting green of its leaves made it an emblem of eternity, for both which reasons they planted it near tombs. In northern England, a relic of this custom is seen in the bearing of rosemary in funeral processions, the sprays being cast on the coffin in the grave. As a plant of remembrance, it formed a part of bridal wreaths. When Christmas was the heartiest of holidays, rosemary decked the hall of feasting, the roast, the boar's head, and the wassail bowl, this service in possible memory of the rosemary's opening to hide the Virgin and her child from Herod's soldiers — a legend it shares with the juniper and other trees. And because Mary spread the linen of her babe on a rosemary, it flowers in memory of him on the day of the passion. In Sicily it is a heathen plant, for fairies nestle under it, disguised as snakes, which circumstance has not prevented its extensive cultivation, even in monastery gardens, where it was prized for its medicinal qualities.

— **Charles Montgomery Skinner,** *Myths and Legends of Flowers, Trees, Fruits and Plants,* **1911**

ROSEMARY 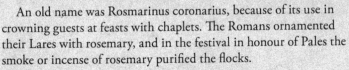 *continued.*

An old name was Rosmarinus coronarius, because of its use in crowning guests at feasts with chaplets. The Romans ornamented their Lares with rosemary, and in the festival in honour of Pales the smoke or incense of rosemary purified the flocks.

(...)

In Herrick's day it was worn at weddings also, hence his apostrophy:

'Grow for two ends, it matters not at all.
Be't for my bridal or my burial.'

We have the note that sprigs of rosemary mingled in the coronal which bound the hair of Anne of Cleves on her nuptial day, and recall how the plant garlanded the wassail bowl of those times, or other Christmas dishes:

'The boar's head in hand bring I
With garlands gay and Rosemary.'

In Germany an old Christmas custom is remembered of demanding presents from women on Good Friday by striking them with sprays of rosemary.

– Marcus Woodward, *How to Enjoy Flowers*, 1928

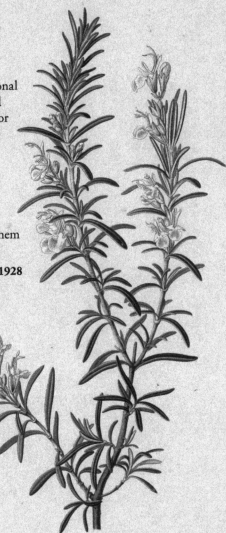

Pl. LV.

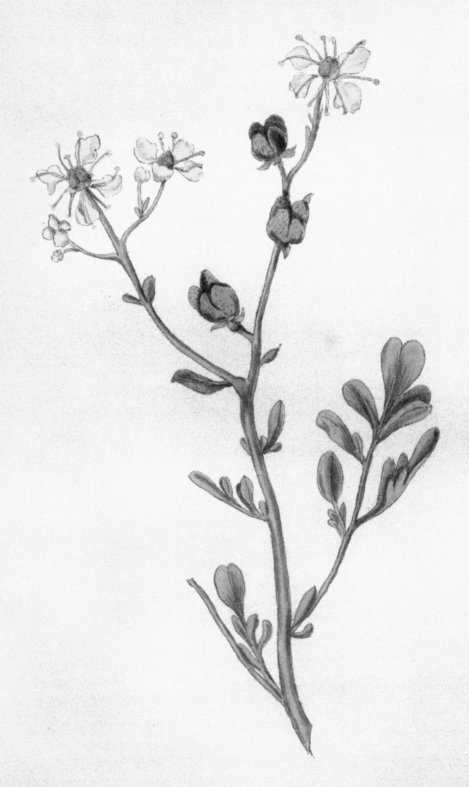

Ruta Graveolens.

A. W. del A. M. Trace. lith.

Tho⁸ Harrild. imp

RUE

Other Names: Herb-of-Grace, Herbygrass, Garden Rue
Latin Name: Ruta graveolens
Symbolises: Fecundity of fields, disgust, disdain
Type: Hardy evergreen shrub
Natural Habitat: Southern Europe
Growing Zone: 4–9
Site: Sunny and dry spot
Sow: April
Harvest: May to June
Usable Parts: Flowers and stem
Companion Plants: Figs, lavender, and raspberries
Herbal Astrology: The Sun

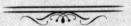

Shrouded in mysticism since antiquity, rue has long been revered as a sacred herb. Once regarded as a potent magical ingredient in spells and charms, now it is often overlooked. Its spray of yellow flowers and evergreen, ferny foliage offers an ornamental dimension to the herb garden. Although it was once a common ingredient in recipes, it is not commonly found in modern cuisine. It should be consumed sparingly, now known to cause gastric discomfort in some people.

One of our oldest and most interesting garden plants and so clustered with lore and traditions that any adequate account of it would fill a small book… Its curious blue-green foliage, as vivid in mid-winter as in summer, its quaintly decorative, albeit small, yellow flowers and its old-world air, all combine to give it a character apart.

– Eleanour Sinclair Rohde, *Herbs and Herb Gardening*, 1936

RUE

continued.

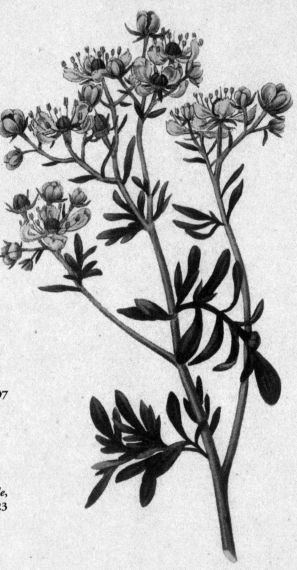

Poor Queen, so that thy state might be no worse,
I would my skill were subject to thy curse.
Here did she fall a tear; here in this place
I'll set a bank of rue, sour herb of grace.
Rue, even for ruth, here shortly shall be seen,
In the remembrance of a weeping queen.

   – **William Shakespeare,** *Richard II*, **Act 4, Scene 4, 1597**

For you there's Rosemary and Rue; these keep
Seeming and savour all the winter long:
Grace and remembrance to you both,...

      – **William Shakespeare,** *A Winter's Tale*,
            Act 4, Scene 3, 1623

Michael from Adam's eyes the film 'emoved
...then purged with euphrasy and rue,
The visual nerve; for he had much to see.

      – **John Milton,** *Paradise Lost*, **1667**

RUE

continued.

I walked alone and thinking,
  And faint the nightwind blew
And stirred on mounds at crossways
  The flower of sinner's rue.

Where the roads part they bury
  Him that his own hand slays,
And so the weed of sorrow
  Springs at the four cross ways.

By night I plucked it hueless,
  When morning broke 'twas blue:
Blue at my breast I fastened
  The flower of sinner's rue.

It seemed a herb of healing,
  A balsam and a sign,
Flower of a heart whose trouble
  Must have been worse than mine.

Dead clay that did me kindness,
  I can do none to you,
But only wear for breastknot
  The flower of sinner's rue.

– A. E. Housman, 'Sinner's Rue', 1922

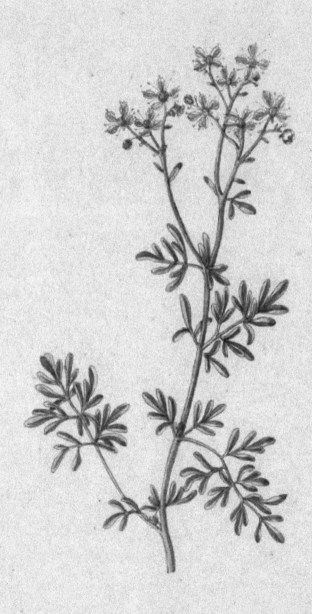

RUE

In the Garden

Rue was introduced into England about the year 1562, and is now cultivated in most gardens, flowering from June to September.

— **George Spratt,** *Flora Medica,* **1829**

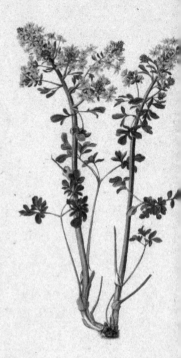

Rue (…) is generally sown while the west winds prevail, as well as just after the autumnal equinox. This plant has an extreme aversion to cold, moisture, and dung; it loves dry, sunny localities, and a soil more particularly that is rich in brick clay; it requires to be nourished, too, with ashes, which should be mixed with the seed as well, as a preservative against the attacks of caterpillars.

— **Elder Pliny,** *The Natural History of Pliny,* **c. 77 AD**

The plant grows almost anywhere, but thrives best in a partially sheltered and dry situation. Propagation may be effected: (1) by seeds, sown outside, broadcast, in spring, raked in and the beds kept free from weeds, the seedlings, when about 2 inches high, being transplanted into fresh beds, allowing about 18 inches each way, as the plants become busy; (2) by cuttings, taken in spring and inserted for a time, until well rooted, in a shady border; (3) by rooted slips, also taken in spring. Every slip or cutting of the young wood will readily grow, and this is the most expeditious way of raising a stock.

Rue will live much longer and is less liable to be injured by frost in winter when grown in a poor, dry, rubbishy soil than in good ground.

— **Maude Grieve,** *A Modern Herbal,* **1931**

In the Kitchen

Green, black or mixed olive relish to be made thus. Remove stones from green, black or mixed olives, then prepare as follows: chop them and add oil, vinegar, coriander, cumin, fennel, rue, mint. Put in a preserving-jar: the oil should cover them. Ready to use.

— **Cato the Elder,** *De Agri Cultura,* **c. 160 BC**

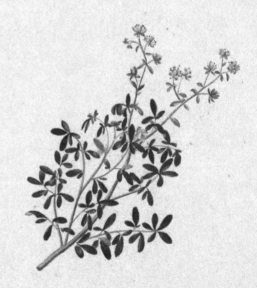

RUE

continued.

ANCIENT KNOWLEDGE, VIRTUES, AND LORE

Medicinal Properties and Remedies

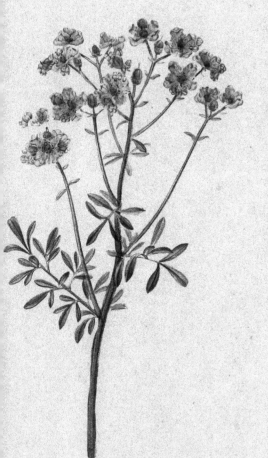

RUE, or Ruta Graveolens, is under the Sun in Leo, therefore will be good for affections of the heart (…) The leaves and the herb are most used in medicine. It is a native of the South of Europe, although it is generally cultivated in this country as a garden shrub. Rue loses much of its activity by drying. Rue tea is a tonic, stimulant, antispasmodic, and emmenagogue.

– Nicholas Culpeper, *Complete Herbal,* **1824**

Rue, herb of grace and memory, stands for repentance also, and we have made the word into a verb, the villain of melodrama assuring the heroine that she will rue the day when she refused to place herself in his power, as she invariably doesn't. It drives away the plague if you merely smell of it; it keeps maids from going wrong in affairs of love, if only they will pause to eat it when tempted; it makes eyes keener and wits more eager; it heals the bites of snakes, scorpions, wasps, and bees. For internal poisons, it seems to have been no less effective than for snake bites; at least, Mithridates, whose subjects were continually trying to poison him, felt a need to accustom his stomach to innutritious material in the faith that if he could not live on it, he could at least keep a-dying for an unconscionable while. And this antidote, which he would take after meals or before a glass, consisted of twenty rue-leaves, two figs, two walnuts, twenty berries of juniper, and a pinch of salt.

– Charles Montgomery Skinner, *Myths and Legends of Flowers, Trees, Fruits and Plants,* **1911**

RUE

continued.

Herbal Magic

The Greeks regarded it as an antimagical herb, because it served to remedy the nervous indigestion they suffered when eating before strangers, which they attributed to witchcraft. In the Middle Ages and later, it was considered - in many parts of Europe - a powerful defence against witches, and was used in many spells. It was also thought to bestow second sight.

> – **Maude Grieve,** *A Modern Herbal,* **1931**

As many stories tell of its powers in divinations. Thus, on the first day of July, a maid who wishes to work a spell should gather a sprig of rosemary, red and white roses, a blue and a yellow flower, a sprig of rue and nine blades of grass, binding them with a hair of her head and sprinkling the nosegay with the blood of a white pigeon. If laid beneath her head when she retires to rest, she will dream of her fate.

> – **Marcus Woodward,** *How to Enjoy Flowers,* **1928**

If you can get a shoe which a girl has worn you may make sad havoc with her heart if you carry it near your own. Also hang it up over your bed and put into it the leaves of rue.

> – **Charles Godfrey Leland,** *Gypsy Sorcery and Fortune Telling,* **1891**

Then there is the love charm of the Love Bag for maidens, by which the Romany chi dreams who her chal shall be. For this they must have the front left foot of a rabbit, three pebbles, a piece of rosemary, a piece of rue, four different kinds of straw, wheat, oats, barley, rye, anything dipped in the blood of a pigeon, all these placed in a bag and never opened and never undone. Then they sleep on it, if on a certain night of the year, say March 21st, the new astrological year, romantically equivalent to your midsummer's night, and the face of their lover is revealed to them.

> – **Gipsy Petulengro,** *A Romany Life,* **1935**

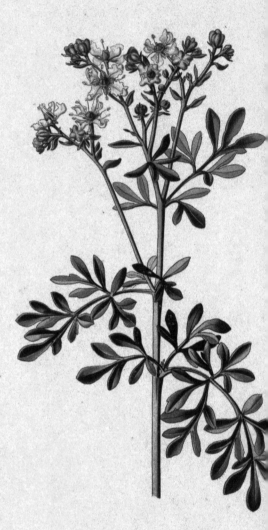

RUE

continued.

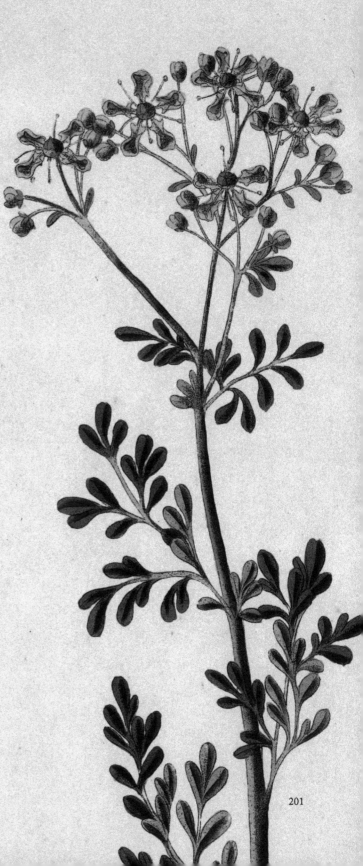

Folk Beliefs

The English herbalists called it Herb Grace and
Serving-men's Joy, because of the multiplicity of
ailments that it was warranted to cure; Mithridates
used the herb as a counterpoison to preserve himself
against infection; and Gerarde records that Serpents
are driven away at the smell of Rue if it be burned,
and that "when the Weesell is to fight with the
Serpent, shee armeth herselfe by eating Rue against
the might of the Serpent."

> **– Richard Folkard,** ***Plant Lore, Legends,***
> ***and Lyrics,*** **1884**

If you pick it you may anticipate a day of family
annoyance; to smell it shows remorse; to carry it
means that you will bear the burdens of others.

> **– Madame Juno,** ***The Gypsy Queen Dream Book and***
> ***Fortune Teller,*** **1930**

Rue was also an antidote to poison, and preserved
people from contagion, particularly that of the
plague, and was though to the of great virtue of
many disorders (...) "It was long, and probably
still is the custom to strew the dock of the Central
Criminal Court at the Old Bailey with Rue. It
arose in 1750, when the contagious disease known
as jail fever, raged in Newgate to a great extent. It
may be remembered that during the trail of the
Manningings (1849), the unhappy woman, after one
of the speeches of the opposing counsel, gathered up
some of the sprigs of Rue which lay before her, and
threw them at his head."

> **– Rosalind Northcote,** ***The Book of Herbs,*** **1903**

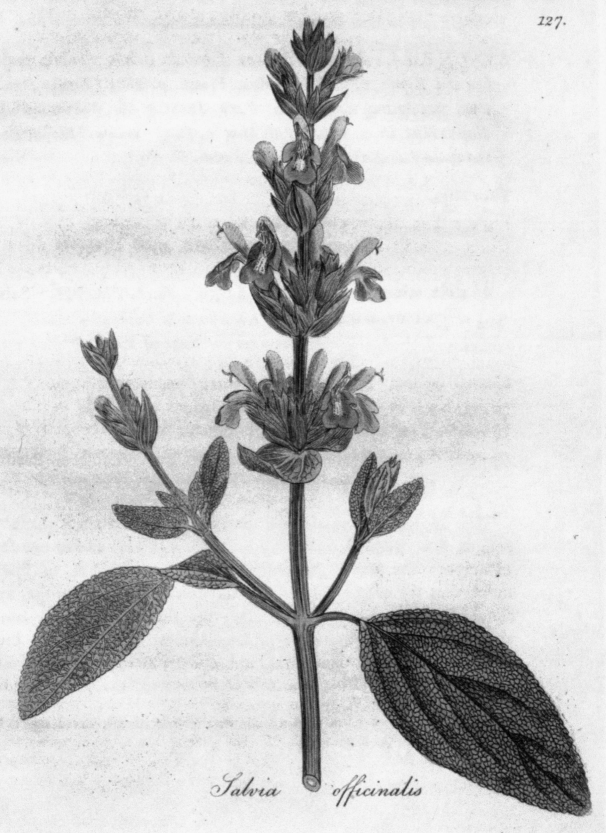

Salvia officinalis

Published by W. Phillips, Feb 1, 1808.

SAGE

Other Names: (Old English) Sawge
Latin Name: Salvia officinalis
Symbolises: Domestic virtue
Type: Perennial, evergreen shrub
Natural Habitat: Northern shores of the Mediterranean
Growing Zone: 4–11
Site: Full sun
Sow: March to April
Harvest: June to August, before flowering
Usable Parts: Leaves and stem
Companion Plants: Fennel, lavender, lemon balm, lemon thyme, lemon verbena, lovage, oregano, parsley, rosemary, savory thyme, and tarragon
Herbal Astrology: Jupiter

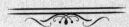

With its beautiful downy leaves, sage is an easy and low-maintenance option to grow in the herb garden. Used either fresh or dried, it is delicious when mixed into stuffings or used to flavour pork dishes. Its delicate purple flowers on spikes are excellent pollinators, making it a favourite among bees and butterflies. It grows particularly well next to herbs like rosemary and oregano.

Few cottage gardens are without this plant, which has been cultivated here for the last three centuries. Gerard in 1596 had it in his garden represented by several varieties. It is not native of England or Northern Europe, but is frequent in warm stony places in the South of France, Spain, Italy, Corsica, Dalmatia, Greece etc. It flowers here in June.

– Robert Bentley, *Medicinal Plants,* **1880**

Sage is for sustenance
 that should man's life sustaine;
For I do stil lie languishing
 continually in paine;
And shall doe still until I die,
 except thou favour show:
My paine and all my grieevous smart,
 ful wel you do it know.

  **– 'A Nosegay Always Sweet, for Lovers to Send for Tokens of Love at
New Year's Tide, or for Fairings', 1584**

In the Garden

Sage can be raised from seed, but it is usually
propagated by cuttings, or layers, or by dividing the
roots. A winter stock of sage-leaves should be secured
by cutting the plants down before they come into
bloom, and then drying them, to be afterwards hung
up in bunches to be used as occasion requires.

  – Isabella Beeton, *Gardening*, 1861

In the Kitchen

Of the use of sage in cookery no special mention need be made. We all know the sage and onion stuffing which appears as the accompaniment of roast pork or duck or goose or other very rich food, but we may not remember that the custom of serving sage with these meats arose from an appreciation of the strongly digestive qualities of the herb. For the same reason in many parts of the country powdered sage is sprinkled over fried onions and occasionally is served with pea soup.

— **Mary Thorne Quelch,** *A Guide to your Herb Garden,* 1951

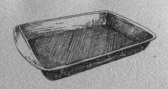

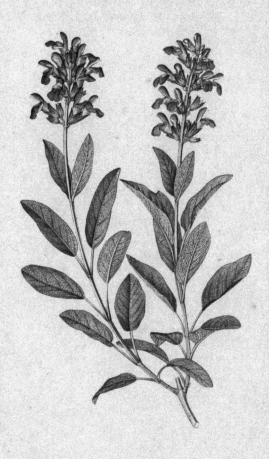

SAGE AND ONION STUFFING.

2 onions,
1 egg,
Little powdered sage,
pepper and salt,
sufficient breadcrumbs to stiffen,
1 oz. butter.

METHOD.

1. Peel and slice onions, and either cook until tender in the butter, leaving the lid on the pan, or boil in water for two hours.

2. Chop onions finely, and, if boiled, add melted butter, sage, pepper, salt, beaten egg, and breadcrumbs to stiffen.

— **H. H. Tuxford,** *Miss Tuxford's Modern Cookery for the Middle Classes,* 1933

ANCIENT KNOWLEDGE, VIRTUES, AND LORE

Medicinal Properties and Remedies

Most of the continental names of the plant are like the botanical one of *Salvia*, from "Salvo", to save or heal, and its high reputation in medicine lasted for ages. The arabians valued it, and the medical school of Salerno summed up its surpassing merits in the line, *Cur morietur homo cui Salvia crescit in horto?* (How can a man die who grows sage in his garden?) Perhaps this originated from the English saying:

'He that would live for aye
Must eat sage in May.'

Parkinson mentions that it is "Much used of many in the month of May fasting," with butter and parsley, and is "held to most" to conduce to health.

– **Rosalind Northcote**, *The Book of Herbs,* **1903**

Sage is singular good for the head and braine; it quickneth the sences and memory, strengthneth the sinews (…) and being put up into the nosthrils, it draweth thin flegme out of the head.

– **John Gerard**, *The Herball; Or, General Historie of Plantes,* **1636**

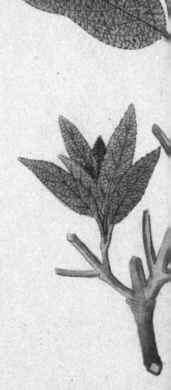

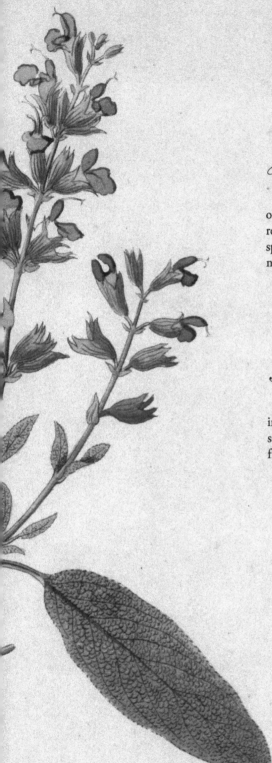

SAGE

Herbal Magic

An ornate variety is the salvia, whose plumes are very flames of scarlet. In the middle ages, when plants were much more remarkable than now, the common sage prolonged life, heightened spirits, kept off toads, enabled girls to see their future husbands, mitigated sorrow, and averted chills.

— **Charles Monthomery Skinner,** *Myths and Legends of Flowers, Trees, Fruits and Plants,* **1911**

Folk Beliefs

It has been claimed that when the Virgin had begun her flight into Egypt she sought refuge from the hunters of Herod in a sage, which she blessed, whereupon the plant put forth a blush of fragrance in all its leaves.

— **Charles Monthomery Skinner,** *Myths and Legends of Flowers, Trees, Fruits and Plants,* **1911**

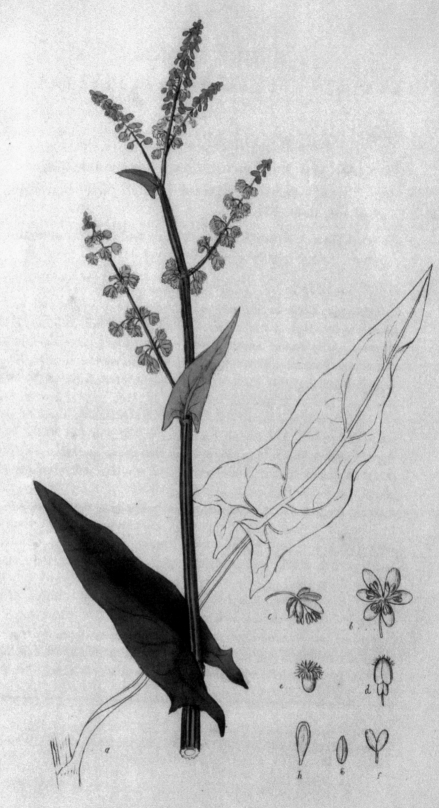

Rumex Acetosa.

Printed by G.E. Madeley 3 Wellington St.

G. Spratt. del. et lith.

SORREL

continued.

Other Names: Garden Sorrel, Common Sorrel
Latin Name: Rumex acetosa
Symbolises: Affection
Type: Hardy Perennial
Natural Habitat: Europe, including Great Britain
Growing Zone: 4–9
Site: Full sun or partial shade
Sow: March to May
Harvest: Two months after planting, from spring through autumn
Usable Parts: Leaves
Companion Plants: Cabbage, strawberries, and tomatoes
Herbal Astrology: Venus

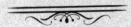

Historically used as a flavouring for sauces, soups, and salads, sorrel's sharp-tasting leaves are now often left out of modern recipes. Garden sorrel works well when planted in a border and provides abundant leaves and small rosette flowers throughout the summer. Pinch out the flower stems to encourage the leaves to grow. The leaves are best picked around 10cm long for eating – add them to your summer salads for an interesting twist.

Of the two kinds of Sorrel cultivated for use as vegetables or salads, Rumex acetosa, the Garden Sorrel, is an indigenous English plant, common, too in the greater part of Europe, in almost all soils and situations. It grows abundantly in meadows, a slender plant about 2 feet high, with juicy stems and leaves, and whorled spikes of reddish-green flowers, which give colour, during the months of June and July, to the grassy spots in which it grows.

It is generally found in pastures where the soil contains iron.

The leaves are oblong, the lower ones 3 to 6 inches in length, slightly arrow-shaped at the base, with very long petioles. The upper ones are sessile. They frequently become a beautiful crimson.

As the flowers increase in size, they become a purplish colour. The stamens and pistils are on different plants. The seeds, when ripe, are brown and shining. The perennial roots run deeply into the ground.

Sorrel is well known for the grateful acidity of its herbage, which is most marked when the plant is in full season, though in early spring it is almost tasteless.

– Maude Grieve, *A Modern Herbal*, 1931

SORREL

White with daisies and red with sorrel
  And empty, empty under the sky!—
Life is a quest and love a quarrel—
  Here is a place for me to lie.

— **Edna St. Vincent Millay, 'Weeds', 1921**

There flourish'd starwort, and the branching beet,
The sorrel acid, and the mallow sweet...

— **William Cowper, 'The Salad. By Virgil', 1799**

In the Garden

Sorrel is a hardy perennial plant. The species as well as the varieties differ to a considerable extent in height and general habit, yet their usage is nearly the same. The finest roots are obtained from seedlings.
    These varieties are propagated by dividing the roots. This method must be adopted in the propagation of the divicious kinds when the male plants are required. All of the varieties will send up a flower-stalk in summer, and it is necessary to cut the stalk when it first develops in order to render the leaves larger and more tender.

— **Jules Arthur Harder,** *The Physiology of Taste,* **1885**

Sown in the spring, sorrel may be cut in the following autumn (…) Sow in drills 9 inches apart, in beds 4 feet wide, covering the seed only slightly with earth; or may be propagated by division of the root.

— **Isabella Beeton,** *Gardening,* **1861**

SORREL

In the Kitchen

Our native species, Rumex acetosa is extremely acid but the cultivated varieties of the Continental species R. scutatus, are better in this respect. The best variety is Oseille large de Belleville, and this is the one recommended for flavouring omelettes or making Sorrel soup. In Brittany fish soups are flavoured with Sorrel, Mint, Parsley, and spring Onions. Before the introduction of French Sorrel our native species was used in cookery and seventeenth and eighteenth-century cookery books contain many recipes (…) folk used to cut up the leaves finely, pound them, and make them into a sauce with vinegar and sugar. Hence the old popular names Green Sauce and Sour Sauce. A little shredded Sorrel is a good addition to salads. John Evelyn said that this herb "imparts so grateful a quickness to the salad that it should never be left out".

— **Eleanour Sinclair Rohde, *Herbs and Herb Gardening*, 1936**

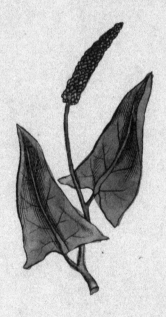

Sorrel Soup.

Wash and trim two pounds of Sorrel, two heads of lettuce and a little chervil, and then cut them in fine shreds. Put them in a saucepan with six ounces of butter, and stir the whole over the fire for twenty-five minutes with a wooden spoon until it is melted. Then add four spoonfuls of flour, and let it cook for ten minutes, stirring it well. (Dilute the flour so there will be no lumps.) Then add in slowly two quarts of boiling water, and as soon as it boils up, set it to one side to boil slowly, and season with salt and pepper. Twenty minutes later add one quart of broth. When it is ready to serve, prepare the following: Dilute a pint of cream with the yolks of four raw eggs; beat it up well, and strain it through a sieve. Add this to the soup with six ounces of butter stirring it well until the butter is melted. Cut two French rolls in fine slices, brown them nicely in the oven, and put them in a soup tureen. Then pour the soup over them and serve.

— **Jules Arthur Harder, *The Physiology of Taste*, 1885**

Sorrel Tart

A Worcestershire lady writes (in 1931) 'In Lancashire they still use the fresh young leaves of wild sorrel (Rumex Acetosa) as a substitute for apple in turnovers. I have made it myself, and very good it is, with plenty of brown sugar and a little moisture on the leaves. Sorrel is in season between apples and gooseberries, i.e. in April and May.'

— **Florence White, *Good Things in England*, 1932**

SORREL

continued.

ANCIENT KNOWLEDGE, VIRTUES, AND LORE

Medicinal Properties and Remedies

COMMON Sorrel, ruled by Venus, grows in gardens as well as fields, and is well known by country-folk. The leaves of Common Sorrel are refrigerant and diuretic; they have an acid taste, and contain binoxalate of potassa and tartaric acid. The juice is excellent against the scurvy. The seeds are astringent, and may be given in powder for flux. The root powdered is also good for purgings, the overflowing of the menses, and bleedings.

Use.—In gravel, itch, jaundice, bilious and putrid fevers, and inflammatory complaints.

Dose.—An infusion of a handful in a quart of water, or boiled in milk in the same proportion to form a whey. Take as much as you like.

– **Nicholas Culpeper & William Joseph Simmonite**, *The Herbal Remedies of Culpeper and Simmonite*, 1957

Folk Beliefs

From May to August the meadows are often ruddy with sorrel, the red leaves of which point out the graves of the Irish rebels who fell on Tara Hill, in the "Ninety-Eight;" the popular and local tradition being that the plants sprang from the blood of the patriots shed on that occasion.

– **Richard Folkard**, *Plant Lore, Legends and Lyrics*, 1884

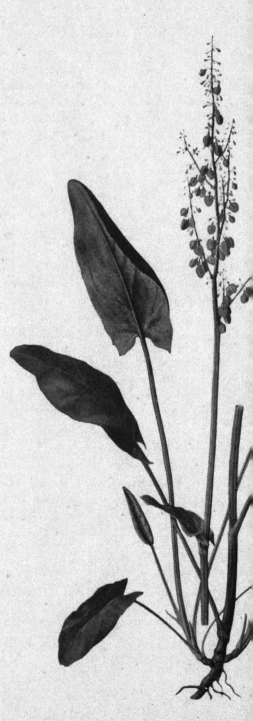

SORREL

continued.

A Witch Story

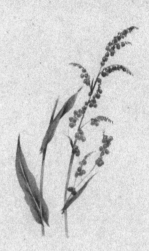

"At Antrim in Ireland a little girl of nineteen (nine?) years of age, inferior to none in the place for beauty, education, and birth, innocently put a leaf of sorrel which she had got from a witch into her mouth, after she had given the begging witch bread and beer at the door; it was scarce swallowed by her, but she began to be tortured in the bowels, to tremble all over, and even was convulsive, and in fine to swoon away as dead. The doctor used remedies on the 9th of May 1698, at which time it happened, but to no purpose, the child continued in a most terrible paroxysm; whereupon they sent for the minister, who scarce had laid his hand upon her when she was turned by the demon in the most dreadful shapes. She began first to rowl herself about, then to vomit needles, pins, hairs, feathers, bottoms of thread, pieces of glass, window-nails, nails drawn out of a cart or coach-wheel, an iron knife about a span long, eggs, and fish-shells and when the witch came near the place, or looked to the house, though at the distance of two hundred paces from where the child was, she was in worse torment, insomuch that no life was expected from the child till the witch was removed to some greater distance. The witch was apprehended, condemned, strangled, and burnt, and was desired to undo the incantation immediately before strangling; but said she could not, by reason others had done against her likewise. But the wretch confessed the same, with many more. The child was about the middle of September thereafter carried to a gentleman's house, where there were many other things scarce credible, but that several ministers and the gentleman have attested the same. The relation is to be seen in a pamphlet printed 1699, and entitled *The Bewitching of a Child in Ireland.*"

(...) The above story, marvellous though it may seem, is capable of explanation. The oxalic acid in sorrel is an irritant poison, causing retching and violent pains. But when once the suspicion of *witchcraft* arose the ejection of such an extraordinary collection of miscellaneous articles followed quite as a matter of course—it would, so to speak, have been altogether against the rules of the game for the girl to have got rid of anything else at that particular date.

— **John D. Seymour,** *Irish Witchcraft and Demonology,* **1913**

Tab. 216

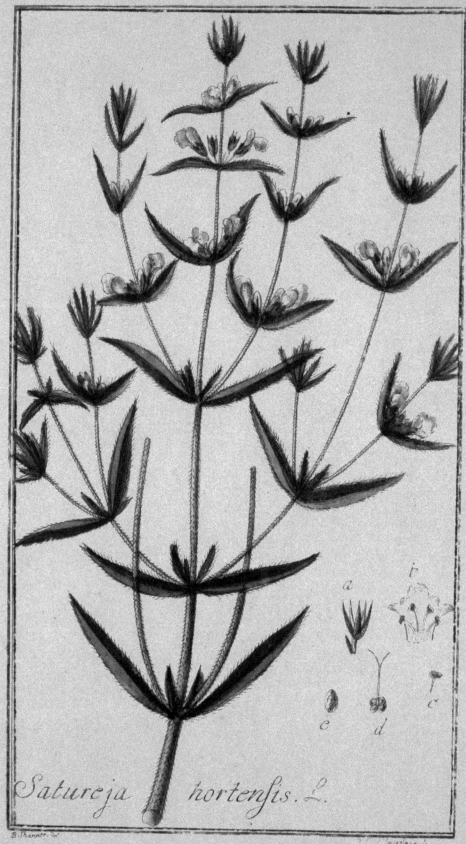

Satureja hortensis. L.

SUMMER SAVORY

Other Names: Bean Herb, Herbe de Sainte Julien
Latin Name: Satureja hortensis
Symbolises: Honesty and sympathy
Type: Annual
Natural Habitat: Europe, including Great Britain
Growing Zone: 5–11
Site: Full sun
Sow: March to April
Harvest: August
Usable Parts: Leaves and stem
Companion Plants: Bergamot and marigolds
Herbal Astrology: Mercury

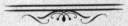

Summer savory is a fragrant herb with ancient roots, once providing aromatic flavour to dishes of old before the arrival of more exotic spices. A key ingredient in the herb mix herbes de Provence, its taste is similar to that of its sibling, winter savoury, although it is less bitter. It flourishes during the warmer months and is best to pick when in flower.

This annual plant has a branching, bushy stem, about eighteen inches in height, woody at the base, frequently changing to purple. The leaves are numerous, small, entire, and acute at the end. The flowers are pink-coloured. It is a native of the south of France. It is extensively cultivated for culinary purposes in Europe and America, and flowers in July and August. The least are the part employed. They have an aromatic odour and taste analogous to those of thyme.

– Oliver Phelps Brown, *The Complete Herbalist*, 1885

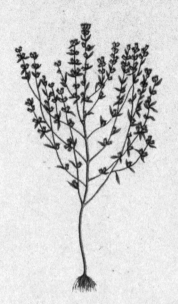

Here's flower for you;
Hot Lavender, Mints, Savory, Marjoram

> **– William Shakespeare,** *A Winter's Tale,*
> **Act 4, Scene 4, 1623**

In the Garden

Summer Savory is an annual. Seed is sown in April in shallow drills a foot apart, the seedlings being thinned to nine inches apart. Full sun and a light, rich soil are essential. The seeds are slow in germinating.

> **– Eleanour Sinclair Rohde,** *Herbs and*
> *Herb Gardening,* **1936**

When the plants have commenced to flower, they should be cut to the ground, tied in small bunches and dried in an airy, shady situation.

> **– Jules Arthur Harder,** *The Physiology of Taste,* **1885**

In the Kitchen

Both Summer Savory (Satureia hortensis) and Winter Savory (Satureia montana) have a strong, very pleasant aromatic flavour, and it is strange that they are not more frequently grown. Before the use of the East Indian spices became common, these two herbs were the most strongly flavoured herbs in use in the kitchen. The date of introduction of Savory into this country is unknown, but the Romans probably introduced both species for they made great use of them in cooking… In France Summer Savory is nearly always boiled with Broad Beans just as we boil Mint with Peas. Either Savory is an excellent ingredient in Lentil soup. Summer and Winter Savory were introduced by the early settlers into America, for they figure in John Josselyn's list.

> **– Eleanour Sinclair Rohde,** *Herbs and*
> *Herb Gardening,* **1936**

The green or dried aromatic tops of the plant are used to mix in stuffing for meat or fowl, in faggots for stews, in salads and with peas and beans. When dried it is sometimes pulverized, and should then be kept in well-stopped vessels. The dried tops are preferred to the green ones for flavoring.

> **– Jules Arthur Harder,** *The Physiology of Taste,* **1885**

ANCIENT KNOWLEDGE, VIRTUES, AND LORE

Medicinal Properties and Remedies

Savory has aromatic and carminative properties, and though chiefly used as a culinary herb, it may be added to medicines for its aromatic and warming qualities. It was formerly deemed a sovereign remedy for the colic and a cure for flatulence, on this account, and was also considered a good expectorant.

– **Maude Grieve**, *A Modern Herbal*, **1931**

To this day country folk know the value of Savory for rubbing on wasp or bee stings.

– **Eleanour Sinclair Rohde**, *Herbs and Herb Gardening*, **1936**

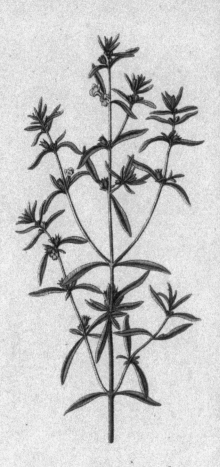

Folk Beliefs

Both species were noticed by Virgil as being among the most fragrant of herbs, and on this account recommended to be grown near bee-hives. There is reason to suppose that they were cultivated in remote ages, before the East Indian spices were known and in common use. Vinegar, flavoured with Savory and other aromatic herbs, was used by the Romans in the same manner as mint sauce is by us.

In Shakespeare's time, Savory was a familiar herb, for we find it mentioned, together with the mints, marjoram and lavender, in *The Winter's Tale*. In ancient days, the Savorys were supposed to belong to the Satyrs, hence the name Satureia. Culpepper says: 'Mercury claims dominion over this herb. Keep it dry by you all the year, if you love yourself and your ease, and it is a hundred pounds to a penny if you do not.'

– **Maude Grieve**, *A Modern Herbal*, **1931**

Plate 116.

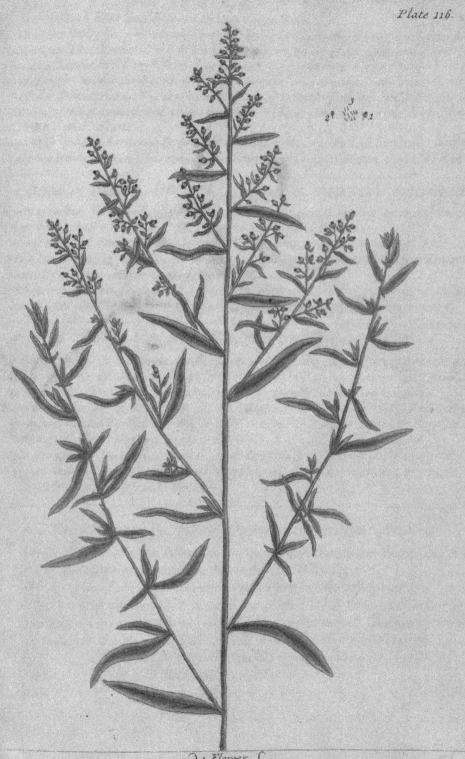

Tarragon.

Eliz.Blackwell delin.sculp.et Pinx.

{ 1. Flower
{ 2. Fruit
{ 3. Seed

{ *Dracunculus hortenfis.*

TARRAGON

Other Names: Dragon, Little Dragon, Mugwort
Latin Name: Artemisia dracunculus
Symbolises: Protection
Type: Hardy herbaceous perennial
Natural Habitat: Siberia
Growing Zone: 4–9
Site: Plant in pots in a sheltered, sunny spot
Sow: April to May
Harvest: May to October
Usable Parts: Leaves and stem
Companion Plants: Chives, lemon balm, lemon thyme, parsley, rosemary, and sage
Herbal Astrology: Mars

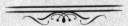

While its name is associated with dragons, its taste is more fragrant than fiery, with a sweet aniseed-like flavour. These days, it's more commonly found in the kitchen than in the medicine cabinet, being a delicious flavouring for chicken or fish. Steep the leaves in hot water for a unique yet calming bedtime tea.

Tarragon is a comparative newcomer in the herb garden, for it was first grown (and then only in the Royal gardens) in Tudor days. Evelyn says that "the tops and young shoots like those of Rocket must never be excluded from sallets. 'Tis highly cordial and friendly to the head, heart, and liver." One old herbalist gives the strange advice that when tarragon is a foot high it should be taken up and put back into the same hole in order to make it grow better!

– Eleanour Sinclair Rohde, *A Garden of Herbs,* **1921**

TARRAGON

continued.

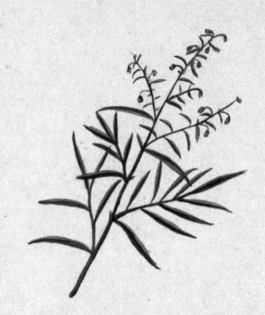

(...) abounding in leisure, fragrant with the scent of the great chestnut-tree, of baskets of raspberries and of a sprig of tarragon.

– **Marcel Proust, 'Overture',** *Swann's Way*, **1922**

In the Garden

The Tarragons like a sandy soil, shelter from cold winds, and though they like a warm spot, they do not object to part shade. They are increased by division in April, and during severe wintry weather the plants should have protection in the form of bracken or litter. They should be planted out two feet apart. Tarragon plants become lanky and worthless after four years and a supply of fresh plants should be maintained.

– **Eleanour Sinclair Rohde,** *Herbs and Herb Gardening*, **1936**

In the Kitchen

Used in making tarragon vinegar. The leaves are sometimes pickled, and sometimes eaten green in salad. A perennial, said to be a native of Siberia, but requires protection in severe weather.

– **Isabella Beeton,** *Gardening*, **1861**

Tarragon Vinegar

Gather the tarragon herb just before it flowers, and on a dry day before the sun has shone on it. Wash it, shake it out of doors, and dry it on a clean cloth. Pick off the leaves, place them in a wide-necked bottle, fill the bottle with the best vinegar, and let it stand for two weeks. Strain through muslin into another bottle, stand uncorked in a saucepan of water reaching almost to the neck, bring the water to the boil, and let it boil for five minutes.

Cork and set aside for use.

Similar vinegar can be made from green mint, horseradish root, garlic, shallots, onions and cucumbers.

– **Marion Neil Harris,** *Beverages, Vinegars and Syrups*, **1914**

TARRAGON *continued.*

ANCIENT KNOWLEDGE, VIRTUES, AND LORE

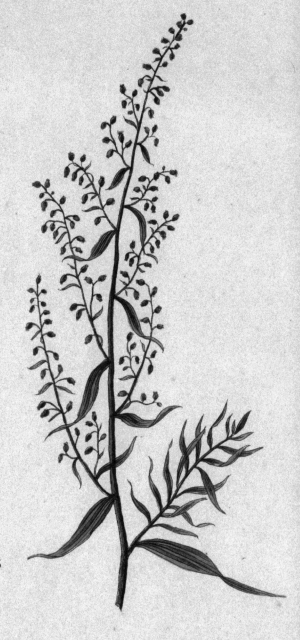

Medicinal Properties and Remedies

'Tis highly cordial and friendly to the Head, Heart, Liver, correcting the weakness of the Ventricle.

— John Evelyn, *Acetaria*, 1699

The root of Tarragon held between the teeth will cure toothache.

— Rosalind Northcote, *The Book of Herbs*, 1903

The Virtues:

Dioscorides writeth, that it is reported that they who have rubbed the leaves or root upon their hands, are not bitten of the viper. Plinie saith, that serpents will not come neere unto him that beareth Dragons around him, and these things are read concerning both the Dragons in the two chapters of Dioscorides. Galen also hath made mention of Dragon in his booke of the faculties of nourishments, where he saith; that the roote of Dragon being twice or thrice sod, to the ende it maye lose all his acrimonie or sharpesse, is sometimes given as Aron or wake-robin is, when it is needfull to expel the more forceably thicke and clammie humours that are troublesome to the chest and lungs. (...) The juice of the garden Dragons, as saith Dioscorides, being dropped into the eies, doth clense them, and greatly amend the dimnesse of the sight.

— **John Gerard**, *The Herball; or, Generall Historie of Plantes*, 1636

Folk Beliefs

The name Tarragon is a corruption of the French Esdragon, derived from the Latin Dracunculus (a little dragon), which also serves as its specific name. It was sometimes called little Dragon Mugwort and in French has also the name Herbe au Dragon. To this, as to other Dragon herbs, was ascribed the faculty of curing the bites and stings of venomous beasts and of mad dogs. The name is practically the same in most countries.

One of the legends told about the origin of Tarragon, which Gerard relates, though without supporting it, is that the seed of flax put into a radish root, or a sea onion, and set in the ground, will bring forth this herb.

— **Maude Grieve**, *A Modern Herbal*, 1931

Tab. 206.

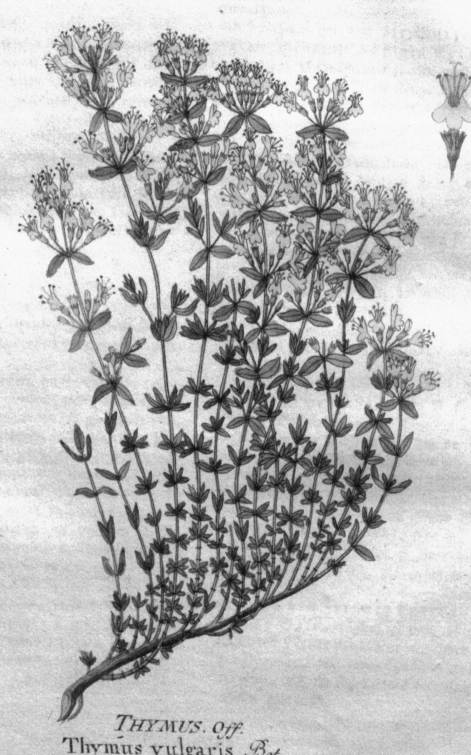

THYMUS. Off.
Thymus vulgaris. Bot.
Der Thymian.

THYME

Other Names: Common Thyme, Garden Thyme
Latin Name: Thymus vulgaris
Symbolises: Spontaneous emotion and activity
Type: Perennial evergreen herb
Natural Habitat: Europe, including Great Britain
Growing Zone: 4–9
Site: Full sun
Sow: March
Harvest: May to June
Usable Parts: Leaves and stem
Companion Plants: Basil, bay, chives, dill, fennel, lavender, lemon verbena, lovage, marjoram, oregano, parsley, rosemary, sage, and savory
Herbal Astrology: Venus

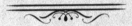

A fragrant favourite of bees, plant thyme among marigolds and nasturtiums for a thriving and colourful garden. Once prized for its medicinal qualities, posies of thyme were worn across Europe as an amulet to protect people from the Black Death. While commonly used in the kitchen to accompany chicken and potato dishes, its essential oil can still be found in some natural anti-inflammatory medicines.

From the Orkneys and far St. Kilda's to the Channel Islands, our native Thyme is one of the loveliest and most fragrant of June and July wild flowers. Thyme and Eye-bright frequently predominate in the exquisite mosaic of minute flowers that carpet chalky uplands, a mosaic to which these flowers contribute their crimson-purple, and pearl. Who can describe the scent of Thyme? A scent so imbued with tonic properties that, like the lark's song, it transports one from this earth into the sunlight and blue heaven above. A scent full of bee-song and honey, of the sunlight of a new-born summer day, and suggestive, as are so many lowly flowers, of all that is pure and sweet, true and strong.

– Eleanour Sinclair Rohde, ***Herbs and Herb Gardening,*** **1936**

THYME

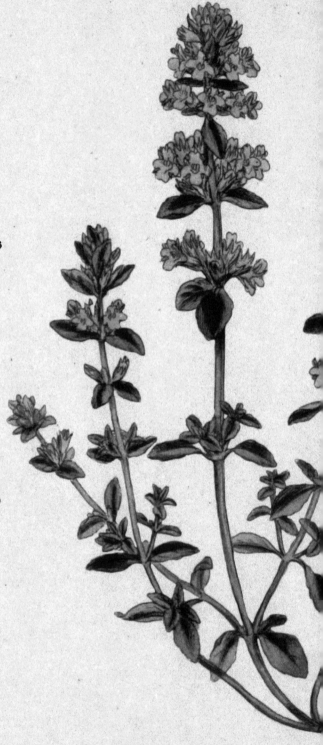

A soft day, thank God!
A wind from the south
With a honeyed mouth;
A scent of drenching leaves,
Briar and beech and lime,
White elder-flower and thyme
And the soaking grass smells sweet,
Crushed by my two bare feet,
While the rain drips,
Drips, drips, drips from the eaves.

– W. M. Letts, 'A Soft Day', 1913

From the forests and highlands
We come we come;
From the river-girt islands,
Where loud waves are dumb
Listening to my sweet pipings.
The wind in the reeds and the rushes,
The bees on the bells of thyme,
The birds of the myrtle bushes,
The cicale above in the lime,
And the lizards below in the grass,
Were as silent as ever old Tmolus was,
Listening to my sweet pipings.

– Percy Bysshe Shelley, 'Hymn of Pan', 1820

What time the mighty moon was gathering light
Love paced the thymy plots of Paradise,
And all about him roll'd his lustrous eyes;
When, turning round a cassia, full in view,
Death, walking all alone beneath a yew,
And talking to himself, first met his sight:
'You must begone,' said Death, 'these walks are mine.'

– Alfred, Lord Tennyson, 'Love and Death', 1830

THYME

continued.

In the Garden

Sow them in April, in shallow drills twelve inches apart. They should be thinned out to eight inches apart, and all weeds should be carefully removed. They may be cut for use as soon as they have made sufficient growth; but for drying, the stalks are gathered as they come into flower.

– **Jules Arthur Harder,** *The Physiology of Taste,* **1885**

The aromatic scent of thyme is very pleasant on a rockery; not only should the silver and golden varieties be grown, but also those bright kinds which give us sheets of purple, pink, and white blossom during summer; to thrive they must be exposed to full sunshine, when they will attract innumerable bees.

– **Violet Biddle,** *Small Gardens and How to Make the Most of Them,* **1901**

All the Thymes like a warm, well-drained soil. On a chalky soil they flourish exceedingly and full sun is essential. The Garden Thymes are propagated either by division of old plants in autumn or spring, or by cuttings taken in early summer. If old plants are not divided they soon show bare patches and become straggly. When raising from seed the seed is planted barely a quarter of an inch deep.

– **Eleanour Sinclair Rohde,** *Herbs and Herb Gardening,* **1936**

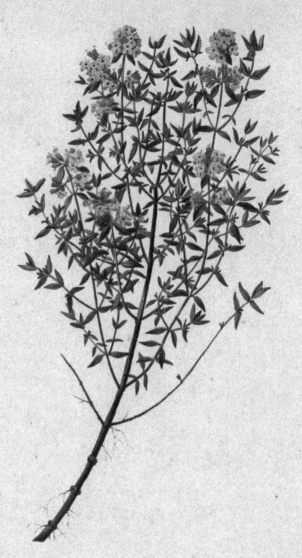

THYME

In the Kitchen

There are two species of Thyme cultivated for culinary purposes: the Common Garden, and the Lemon or Evergreen Thyme, both of which are hardy perennial plants, having a shrubby character and a comparatively long growth. The leaves have an agreeable, aromatic taste, and are used for flavoring soups, stuffings and sauces. They should be used with moderation, as too much imparts a bitter taste to the substance.

— **Jules Arthur Harder,** *The Physiology of Taste,* **1885**

English Herb Chutney

Ingredients

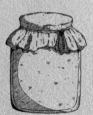

    500g cooking apples (or pears)
    150g soft, dark sugar
    300ml cider vinegar
    1 sprig of thyme (finely chopped leaves)
    1 sprig of rosemary (finely chopped leaves)
    1 lemon (zested)
    1 clove of garlic

Method

1. Core, peel and roughly chop the apples.

2. Place the apples into a large, heavy-bottomed saucepan. Add the chopped thyme, rosemary, garlic and the lemon zest.

3. Bring the temperature up, and cook the ingredients on a medium boil for a couple of minutes.

4. Then, allow to simmer for roughly thirty minutes. Or until the apples (or pears) are nice and soft. The mixture should obtain a thick, 'jam' like consistency.

5. If sufficiently cooked, remove from the heat and allow to cool slightly.

6. Transfer your warm herb chutney into warm sterilised jars. Cover with a wax paper disc and seal.

— **Two Magpies Publishing,** *The A-Z of Homemade Chutneys, Pickles, and Relishes,* **2014**

THYME

continued.

ANCIENT KNOWLEDGE, VIRTUES, AND LORE

Medicinal Properties and Remedies

The oil of thyme is a useful and powerful local stimulant, and may be applied to a carious tooth by means of lint or cotton to relieve toothache; or when mixed with olive oil or spirit, especially if combined with camphor, as a stimulating liniment in chronic rheumatism, sprains, bruises. The chief consumption of oil of thyme, is, however, in veterinary practice. Oil of thyme is also used for scenting soaps.

– **Robert Bentley,** *Medicinal Plants,* **1880**

The essential oil of common thyme was (and is) utilised as a powerful antiseptic and antifungal. Before the advent of modern antibiotics, oil of thyme was additionally used to medicate bandages.

– **David Ellis,** *Medicinal Herbs and Poisonous Plants,* **1918**

Thyme is efficacious as a remedy for the stings of serpents (…) also for the sting of the scolopendra*, both sea and land, the leaves and branches being boiled for the purpose in wine. Burnt, it puts to flight all venomous creatures by its smell, and it is particularly beneficial as an antidote to the venom of marine animals.

– **Elder Pliny,** *The Natural History of Pliny,* **c. 77 AD**

*giant centipede.

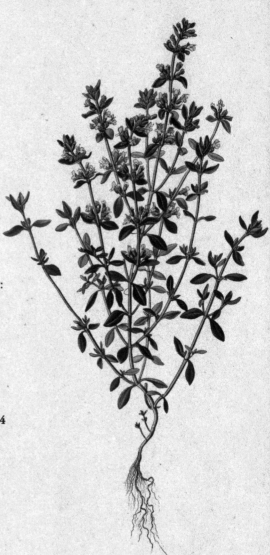

Herbal Magic

In olden times, it was believed that Thyme renewed the spirits of both man and beast; and the old herbalists recommended it is a powerful aid in melancholic and splenetic diseases.—Fairies and elves were reputed to be especially fond of Wild Thyme. Oberon exclaims with delight:—

"I know a bank whereon the Wild Thyme blows,
Where Oxlips and the woody Violet grows,
Quite over-canopied with lush Woodbine.
With sweet Musk-Roses, and with Eglantine."

The fairy king's musical hounds would willingly forsake the richest blossoms of the garden in order to hunt for the golden dew in the flowery tufts of Thyme. Of witches it is said, that when they:

"Won't do penance for their crime,
They bathed themselves in Oregano and Thyme."

(...)

A bunch of wild Thyme and Origanum, laid by the milk in a dairy, prevents its being spoiled by thunder

– Richard Folkard, *Plant Lore, Legends and Lyrics,* 1884

THYME

continued.

Folk Beliefs

The name Thyme, in its Greek form, was first given to the plant by the Greeks as a derivative of a word which meant 'to fumigate,' either because they used it as incense, for its balsamic odour, or because it was taken as a type of all sweet-smelling herbs. Others derive the name from the Greek word thumus, signifying courage, the plant being held in ancient and mediaeval days to be a great source of invigoration, its cordial qualities inspiring courage… Pliny tells us that, when burnt, it puts to flight all venomous creatures.

Among the Greeks, Thyme denoted graceful elegance; 'to smell of Thyme' was an expression of praise, applied to those whose style was admirable. It was an emblem of activity, bravery and energy, and in the days of chivalry it was the custom for ladies to embroider a bee hovering over a sprig of Thyme on the scarves they presented to their knights.

– Maude Grieve, *A Modern Herbal,* **1931**

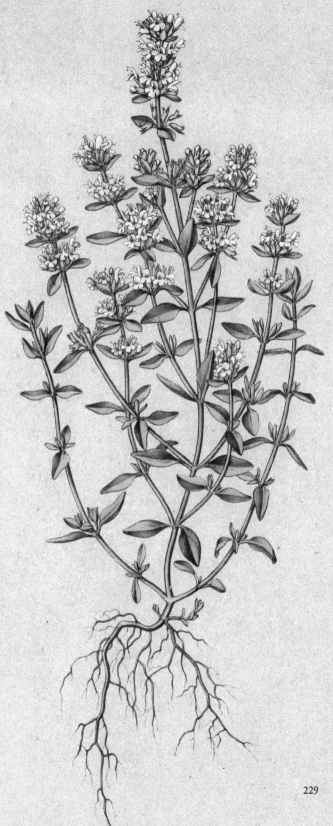

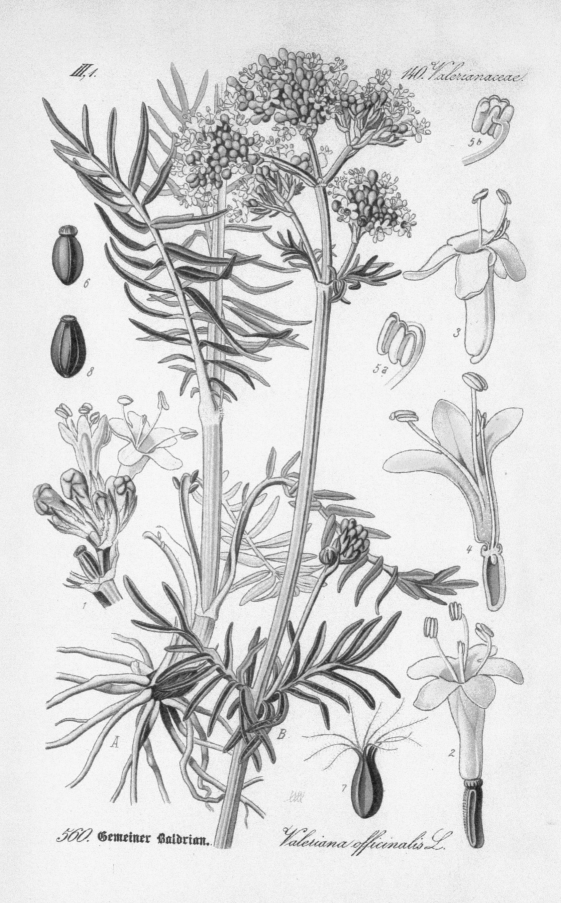

III, 1.   140. *Valerianaceae.*

560. Gemeiner Baldrian.   *Valeriana officinalis L.*

VALERIAN

Other Names: Garden Valerian, Garden Heliotrope, Setwall and All-Heal, Cat's Love, Phu (Gale), Great Wild Valerian, Amantilla, and Setewale Capon's Tail.
Latin Name: Valeriana officinalis
Symbolises: An accommodating disposition
Type: Perennial
Natural Habitat: Europe and Asia
Growing Zone: Zones 4–9
Site: Sun and partial shade, in moist soil
Sow: March to April
Harvest: September to October
Usable Parts: Root
Companion Plants: Catnip, echinacea, dill, oregano, and thyme
Herbal Astrology: Mercury

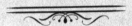

Valerian's dainty clusters of pink and white flowers add a lofty charm to any herb garden and are a key attraction for bees and other pollinators. While also being pleasing on the eye, it is hailed mostly for the virtues of its root, being a common supplement for those looking for a peaceful night's sleep. For an effective night time brew, a sleepy tea can be made from steeping the dried root in freshly boiled water. Due to its sedative properties, consumption of valerian should be avoided during pregnancy.

The plant is found throughout Europe and Northern Asia, and is common in England in marshy thickets and on the borders of ditches and rivers, where its tall stems may generally be seen in the summer towering above the usual herbage, the erect, sturdy growth of the plant, the rich, dark green of the leaves, their beautiful form, and the crowning masses of light-coloured flowers, making the plant conspicuous.

(…)

The flowers are in bloom from June to September. They are small, tinged with pink and flesh colour, with a somewhat peculiar, but not exactly unpleasant smell. The corolla is tubular, and from the midst of its lobes rise the stamens, only three in number, though there are five lobes to the corolla. The limb of the calyx is remarkable for being at first inrolled and afterwards expanding in the form of a feathery pappus, which aids the dissemination of the fruit. The fruit is a capsule containing one oblong compressed seed. Apart from the flowers, the whole plant has a foetid smell, much accentuated when bruised.

– Maude Grieve, *A Modern Herbal,* **1931**

VALERIAN

continued.

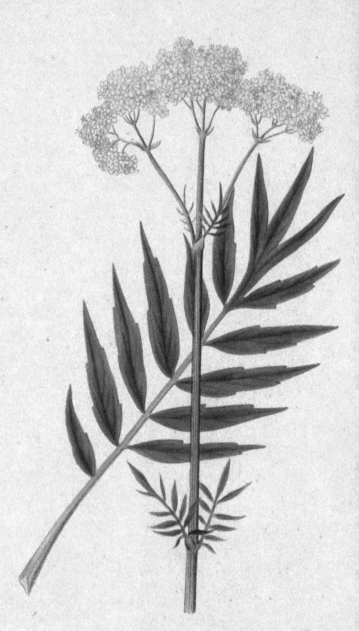

Broken, bewildered by the long retreat
  Across the stifling leagues of southern plain,
  Across the scorching leagues of trampled grain,
Half-stunned, half-blinded, by the trudge of feet
And dusty smother of the August heat,
  He dreamt of flowers in an English lane,
  Of hedgerow flowers glistening after rain—
All-heal and willow-herb and meadow-sweet.

All-heal and willow-herb and meadow-sweet—
  The innocent names kept up a cool refrain—
All-heal and willow-herb and meadow-sweet,
  Chiming and tinkling in his aching brain,
  Until he babbled like a child again—
"All-heal and willow-herb and meadow-sweet."

    – Wilfrid Wilson Gibson, 'Retreat', 1915

...The maiden in a morn betime,
Went forth when May was in the prime.
  To get sweet setywall,
    The honeysuckle, the harlock,
    The lily and the ladysmock,
To deck her summerhall.

    – Michael Drayton, 'Eclogue', 1593

VALERIAN

continued.

In the Garden

Valerian is a pretty herb but a rampant grower, and on good soil attains quite four feet.

> – **Eleanour Sinclair Rohde,** *Herbs and Herb Gardening,* **1936**

Valerian does well in all ordinary soils, but prefers rich, heavy loam, well supplied with moisture.

> – **Maude Grieve,** *A Modern Herbal,* **1931**

Young flowering wild plants which develop at the end of slender runners that are given off by the perennial runners, are usually chosen for transplanting. These are planted on land treated with farmyard manure. It is advantageous to give plenty of liquid manure and artificial manure from time to time. The plants are also given plenty of water. As only the rhizomes are collected, the flowering tops are cut off as much as possible in order to encourage the growth of the rhizome. In September or October the tops are cut off with a scythe, and the rhizomes allowed to be dug up. These are sliced longitudinally to facilitate washing, washed thoroughly, and dried on a shed floor about 6 feet from the ground. The wet material is strewn on perforated boards, below which a large coke stove is kept going until the drying is complete. About 24 parts of the dry product are obtained from 100 parts of fresh rhizomes.

> – **David Ellis,** *Medicinal Herbs and Poisonous Plants,* **1918**

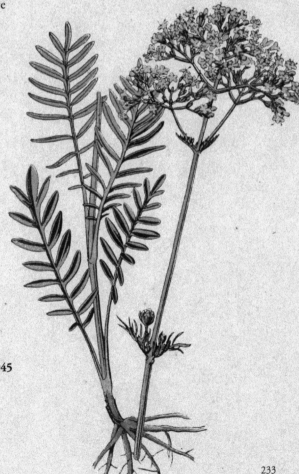

The small, pale pink flowers of the wild valerian are commonly visited by bees for nectar. The plant is often to be found in damp shady places near streams and should not be confused with the red valerian (*Kentranthus ruber*) of the flower garden which is naturalized in many areas, for this plant has too long a flower tube to be of any use to the hive bee.

> – **Frank N. Howes,** *Plants and Beekeeping,* **1945**

VALERIAN

continued.

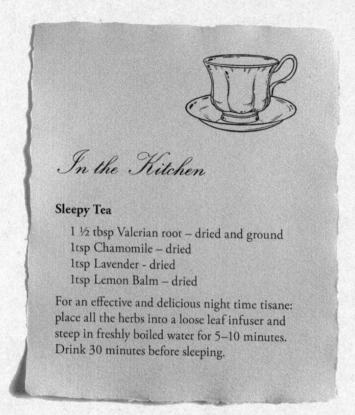

In the Kitchen

Sleepy Tea

1 ½ tbsp Valerian root – dried and ground
1tsp Chamomile – dried
1tsp Lavender - dried
1tsp Lemon Balm – dried

For an effective and delicious night time tisane:
place all the herbs into a loose leaf infuser and
steep in freshly boiled water for 5–10 minutes.
Drink 30 minutes before sleeping.

ANCIENT KNOWLEDGE, VIRTUES AND LORE

Medicinal Properties and Remedies

In medicine, the root of V. officinalis is intended when Valerian is mentioned. It is supposed to be the Phu (an expression of aversion from its offensive odour) of Dioscorides and Galen, by whom it is extolled as an aromatic and diuretic.

– **Maude Grieve,** *A Modern Herbal,* **1931**

VALERIAN is under the dominion of Uranus. It is good for fits, and will exert its influence on the nervous system, first as a stimulant, and then a sedative, but it is not a narcotic. There are two kinds of Valerian, the garden Valerian and the wild Valerian. The wild is the best, and the root is the part used in medicine.

– **Nicholas Culpeper & William Joseph Simmonite,** *Herbal Remedies of Culpeper and Simmonite,* **1957**

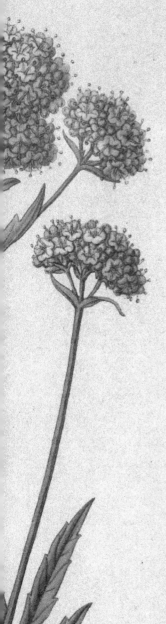

VALERIAN *continued.*

During the recent War, when air-raids were a serious strain on the overwrought nerves of civilian men and women, Valerian, prescribed with other simple ingredients, taken in a single dose, or repeated according to the need, proved wonderfully efficacious, preventing or minimizing serious results.

– **Maude Grieve**, *A Modern Herbal*, 1931

The leaves were used to make an ointment for wounds; the roots were regarded as a remedy for the Plague and from very ancient times Valerian was regarded as a specific for nervous complaints. The dried roots of Valerian have a strong and rather unpleasant odour, but this odour was much appreciated in past centuries and Turner states in his Herbal that the roots were laid amongst clothes to perfume them.

– **Eleanour Sinclair Rohde**, *Herbs and Herb Gardening*, 1936

If you wet lint in the juice of valerian, & put it into any wound, made either with arrow, or sword, or otherwise, and the drosse or grosse part thereof laide upon it, you shall cause the iron to come forth if any such be staid behinde, and so also heale the wound.

– **Marcus Woodward**, *The Countryman's Jewel –Days in the Life of a Sixteenth-Century Squire*, 1934

The dry root is put into counterpoysons and medicines preservative against the pestilence: whereupon it hath been had (and is to this day among the poore people of our Northerne parts) in such veneration amongst them, that no broths, pottage or physicall meats are worth any thing, if Setwall were not at an end: whereupon some upon some woman Poet or other hath made these verses.

'They that will have their heale,
Must put Setwall in their keale.'

– **John Gerard**, *The Herball; or, Generall Historie of Plantes*, 1636

VALERIAN

continued.

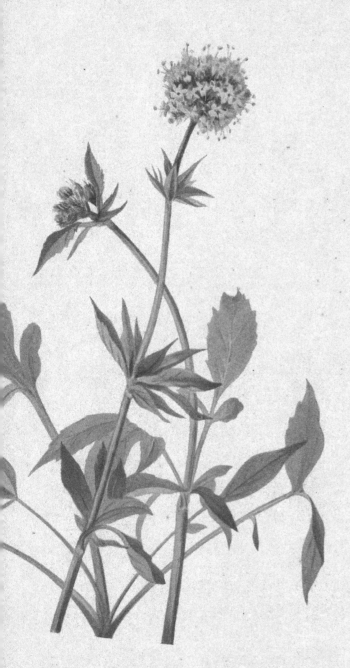

Herbal Magic

Make unto thyself a Sprinkler of vervain, fennel, lavender, sage, valerian, mint, garden-basil, rosemary, and hyssop, gathered in the day and hour of Mercury, the moon being in her increase. Bind together these herbs with a thread of a young maiden, and engrave [figures] upon the handle...

After this thou mayest use the Water, using the Sprinkler whenever it is necessary; and know that wheresoever thou shalt sprinkle this Water, it will chase away all Phantoms, and they shall be unable to hinder or annoy any.

— **S. Liddell Macgregor Mathers**, *The Key of Solomon the King*, 1889

Dioscorides accounteth... wilde Hemp, and Valerian, hung up in the house, an amulet against witchcraft.

— **John Baptista Porta**, *Natural Magick*, 1558

Folk Beliefs

Among the simple country folks, even at the present day, a bridegroom stands in dread of the envy of the Elves, to counteract which it has long been a custom to lay in the clothes on the wedding day certain strong-smelling plants, as garlic or valerian. Near gates and in crossways there is supposed to be the greatest danger.

— **Benjamin Thorpe**, *Northern Mythology*, 1851

The root of the herb valerian (called Phu), is very like to the eye of a cat, and wheresoever it groweth, if cats come thereunto, they instantly dig it up for the love thereof, as I myself have seen in mine own garden, for it smelleth moreover like a cat.

— **Edward Topsell**, *The History of Four-Footed Beasts and Serpents*, 1658

VALERIAN

continued.

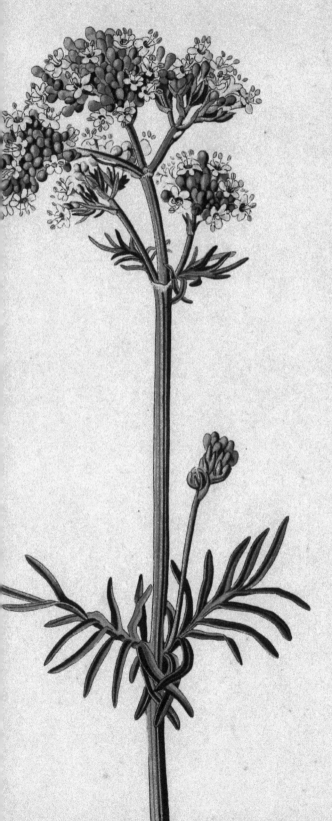

It has been suggested that the famous Pied Piper of Hamelin owed his irresistible power over rats to the fact that he secreted Valerian roots about his person.

> **– Maude Grieve,** *A Modern Herbal,* **1931**

If a maiden wears valerian in her girdle or her corsets, she will attract the opposite sex.—Wales.

> **– M. A. Radford & E. Radford,** *Encyclopaedia of Superstitions – A History of Superstition,* **1947**

To Attract Bees.

Gather foxglove, raspberry leaves, wild marjorum, mint, camomile, and valerian; mix them with butter made on May Day, and let the herbs also be gathered on May Day. Boil them all together with honey; then rub the vessel into which the bees should gather, both inside and out, with the mixture; place it in the middle of a tree, and the bees will soon come.

> **– Jane Wilde,** *Ancient Legends, Mystic Charms and Superstitions of Ireland,* **1919**

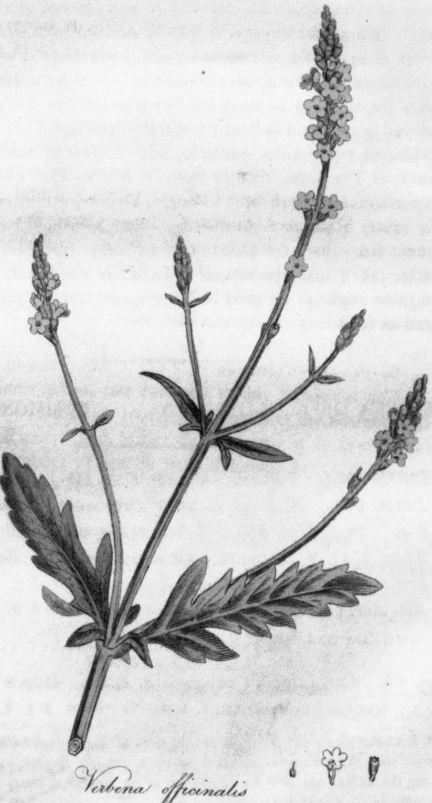

Verbena officinalis

Published by W. Phillips, March 1 1808.

VERBENA

Other Names: Vervain, Simpler's Joy, Holy Herb
Latin Name: Verbena officinalis
Symbolises: Enchantment, energy in adversity, you have my confidence
Type: Hardy herbaceous perennial
Natural Habitat: South and North America and Europe
Growing Zone: 8–11
Site: Full sun
Sow: February to May
Harvest: May to September
Usable Parts: Flowers, leaves, and stem
Companion Plants: Coriander, dill, and garlic
Herbal Astrology: Venus

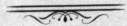

With its age-old associations with the divine and supernatural, verbena has been a common ingredient in religious rituals and divinatory practices. Not so much a culinary herb, this enchanting plant is a delight to grow in the herb garden, with its tall, architectural clusters of purple flowers providing structure and colour to any bed. Favouring warm and sunny conditions, its fragrant blooms are now regarded as a valuable pollinator for butterflies.

The common Vervain hath somewhat long broad leaves next the ground deeply gashed about the edges, and some only deeply dented, or cut all alike, of a blackish green colour on the upper side, somewhat grey underneath. The stalk is square, branched into several parts, rising about two feet high, especially if you reckon the long spike of flowers at the tops of them, which are set on all sides one above another, and sometimes two or three together, being small and gaping, of a blue colour and white intermixed, after which come small round seed, in small and somewhat long heads. The root is small and long. It grows generally throughout this land in divers places of the hedges and way-sides, and other waste grounds.

– Nicholas Culpeper, *Complete Herbal,* 1824

VERBENA

Vervain and dill
Hinders witches from their will.

— **John Aubrey,** *Miscellanies upon Various Subjects,* **1721**

Hallowed be thou, Vervain,
As thou growest on the ground,
For in the Mount of Calvary,
There thou wast first found.
Thou healedst our Saviour Jesus Christ,
And staunchedst his bleeding wound;
In the name of the Father, Son, and Holy Ghost,
I take thee from the ground.

— **John Harland & Thomas Turner Wilkinson,**
Lancashire Folk-Lore, **1867**

In the Garden

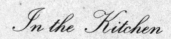

Although a perennial, it wants treating like a snapdragon—sown in gentle heat in February, thinned, pricked off, hardened in a frame, and planted out in May. Plants thus treated will be in full bloom in July, and they will keep on growing and flowering for many weeks. One can buy mixed seed, or separate colours, such as purple, blue, scarlet, pink and white, and striped. Many of the dark flowers have a white eye. It is not wise to give too rich a soil, or the plants will straggle; in any case it may be found necessary to peg them down.

— **Walter P. Wright,** *The Perfect Garden – How to Keep it Beautiful and Fruitful,* **1909**

In the Kitchen

A fresh geranium or lemon verbena leaf gives a delightful odor and taste to jelly.

— **Anon,** *Vaughan's Vegetable Cook Book,* **1919**

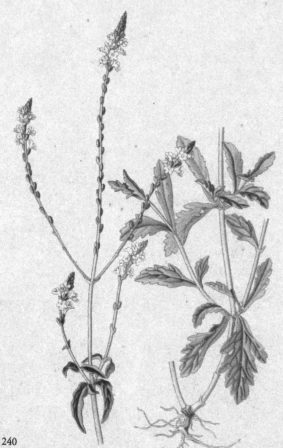

VERBENA

continued.

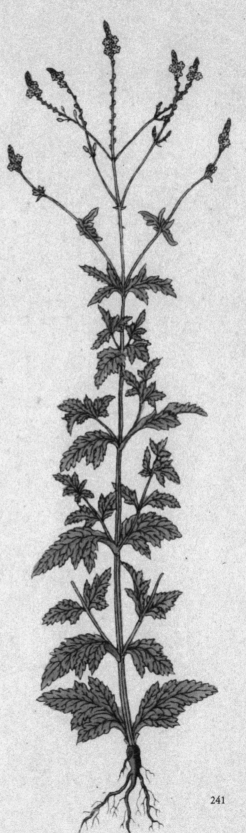

ANCIENT KNOWLEDGE, VIRTUES, AND LORE

Medicinal Properties and Remedies

Hot and dry, a great opener, cleanser, healer, it helps the yellow jaundice, defects in the reins and bladder, pains in the head; if it be but bruised and hung about the neck, all diseases in the privities; made into an ointment it is a sovereign remedy for old head-aches, as also frenzies, it clears the skin, and causes a lovely colour.

— **Nicholas Culpeper,** *Complete Herbal,* **1824**

It is asserted, that the most acute and obstinate head-achs have been removed by the use of vervain, both internally in the form of a decoction, and also by suspending the herb round the neck.

— **Anthony Florian Madinger Willich,** *Domestic Encyclopædia,* **1802**

Vervain is under Venus, and will strengthen the womb. It grows wild in many places by the wayside, and flowers in July.

Infusion of Vervain.—3 ounces of the fresh tops of Vervain, 1 ounce of raspberry leaves, and 1 ounce of pennyroyal, to 1 quart of water; a little ginger and sugar may be added.

Dose.—A wineglassful three times a day.

Use.—Obstructions of liver and spleen, nervousness, smallpox, wheezing, scurvy, worms, gravel, and stoppage of urine.

— **Nicholas Culpeper & William Joseph Simmonite,** *The Herbal Remedies of Culpeper and Simmonite,* **1957**

VERBENA

Herbal Magic

The Vervain, or Verbena, has from time immemorial been the symbol of enchantment, and the most ancient nations employed this plant in their divinations, sacrificial and other rites, and in incantations. It bore the names of the Tears of Isis, Tears of Juno, Mercury's Blood, Persephonion, Demetria, and Cerealis. The Magi of the ancient Elamites or Persians made great use of the Vervain in the worship of the Sun, always carrying branches of it in their hands when they approached the altar. The magicians also employed the mystic herb in their pretended divinations, and affirmed that, by smearing the body over with the juice of this plant, the person would obtain whatever he set his heart upon, and be able to reconcile the most inveterate enemies, make friends with whom he pleased, and gain the affections, and cure the disease of whom he listed. When they cut Vervain, it was always at a time when both sun and moon were invisible, and they poured honey and honeycomb on the earth, as an atonement for robbing it of so precious a herb.

The Greeks called it the Sacred Herb, and it was with this plant only that they cleansed the festival-table of Jupiter before any great solemnity took place; and hence, according to Pliny, the name of Verbena is derived. It was, also, one of the plants which was dedicated to Venus. Venus Victrix wore a crown of Myrtle interwoven with Vervain.— With the Romans, the Vervain was a plant of good omen, and considered strictly sacred:—

"Bring your garlands, and with reverence place
The Vervain on the altar."

They employed it in their religious rites, swept their temples and cleansed their altars with it, and sprinkled holy water with its branches. They also purified their houses with it, to keep off evil spirits; and in order to make themselves invulnerable, they carried about their persons a blade of Grass and some Vervain. Their ambassadors, or heralds-at-arms, wore crowns of Vervain when they went to offer terms of reconciliation, or to give defiance to their enemies, a custom thus noticed by Drayton:—

"A wreath of Vervain heralds wear,
   Amongst our garlands named;
Being sent that dreadful news to bear,
   Offensive war proclaimed."

– **Richard Folkard,** *Plant Lore, Legends and Lyrics,* **1884**

Two of those most frequently used as ingredients in the mystic caldron were the vervain and the rue, these plants having been specially credited with super-natural virtues. (...) Although vervain, therefore, as the "enchanters' plant," was gathered by witches to do mischief in their incantations, yet, as Aubrey says, it "hinders witches from their will," a circumstance to which Drayton further refers when he speaks of the vervain as "'gainst witchcraft much avayling."

– **Thomas Firminger Thiselton Dyer,** *Plants in Witchcraft,* **1889**

VERBENA

continued.

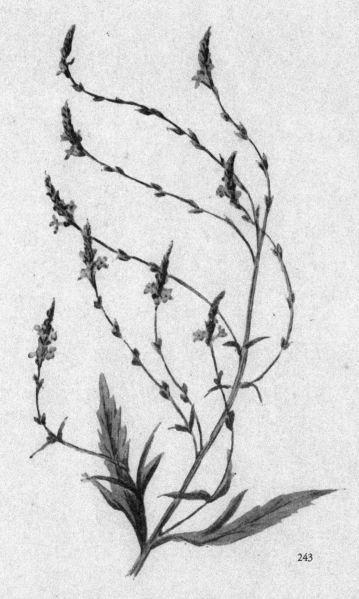

Folk Beliefs

Bruised, it was worn round the neck as a charm against headaches, and also against snake and other venomous bites as well as for general good luck. It was thought to be good for the sight. Its virtues in all these directions may be due to the legend of its discovery on the Mount of Calvary, where it staunched the wounds of the crucified Saviour. Hence, it is crossed and blessed with a commemorative verse when it is gathered. It must be picked before flowering, and dried promptly.

– Maude Grieve, *A Modern Herbal,* **1931**

Vervain was one of the herbs held most sacred by the Druids and, as the herbals of Gerard and Parkinson testify, it was in high repute even as late as the sixteenth and seventeenth centuries. It has never been satisfactorily identified, though many authorities incline to the belief that it was verbena. In Druidical times libations of honey had to be offered to the earth from which it was dug, mystic ceremonies attended the digging of it and the plant was lifted out with the left hand. This uprooting had always to be performed at the rising of the dog star and when neither the sun nor the moon was shining.

– Eleanour Sinclair Rohde, *The Old English Herbals,* **1922**

243

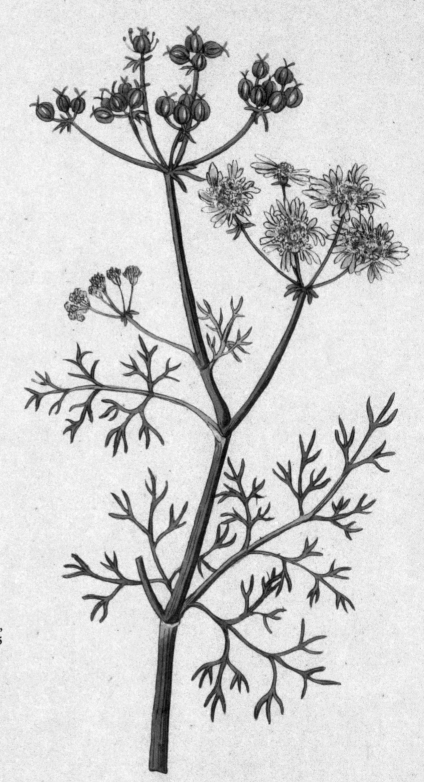

Thus ends in brief,
of herbs the chief,
To get more skill,
Read whom ye will;
Such mo to have,
Of field go crave.

**– Wilfrid Wilson Gibson,
'Retreat', 1915**

GLOSSARY

Ague – An intermitting fever, with cold fits succeeded by hot; the cold fit is, in popular language, more particularly called the ague; and the hot, the fever.

Almanac(k) – A calendar; a book in which the revolutions of the seasons, with the turn of feasts and fasts, is noted for the ensuing year.

Annual – That which only lasts a year. In this instance, the word refers to plants that complete their life cycle within a single growing season.

Aperient – Laxative – has the quality of opening; chiefly used in medicines, gently purgative.

Asp – A kind of serpent, whose poison kills without possibility of apply any remedy.

Biennial – Of the continuance of two years. Plants that flower and seed again in their second growing season.

Carminative – [supposed to be so called, as having *vim carminis*, the power of a charm.] Carminatives are such things as dilute and relax at the same time, because wind occasions a spasm, or convulsion in some parts. Whatever promotes insensible perspiration, is carminative; for wind is perspirable matter retained in the body.

Calyx – The outer envelope of a flower.

Cephalic – That which is medicinal to the head.

Corolla – The coloured part of a flower, composed of a petal or petals. The term is only applied when the calyx is present, otherwise it is called a perianth.

Decoction – The act of boiling anything, to extract its virtues.

Defluxion – The flow of humours downward.

Diaphoretic – *Sudorifick*; promoting a diaphoresis or perspiration; causing sweat.

Discutient – A medicine that has power to dispel or drive back the matter of tumours in the blood. It sometimes means the same as carminative.

Diuretic – Having the power to provoke urine.

Doctrine – The principles or positions of any sect or master; that which is taught.

Drachms (or dram) – The eighth part of an ounce.

Dyspepsia – [Dyspepy] A difficulty of digestion, or bad fermentation in the stomach or guts.

Effusion – The act of pouring out.

Emetic(k) – The quality of provoking vomits.

Emmenagogue – Medicines that promote the menstrual courses, either by giving a greater force to the blood in its circulation, or by making it thinner.

Emollient – Such things as sheath and soften the asperities of the humours, and relax and supple the solids at the same time.

Exanthema – [Examthemata] A skin rash.

Expectorant – A medicine which promotes expectoration. [*Expectorate* – Of a drug or its action: To clear or drive out (phlegm, etc) from the chest or lungs.]

Fomentations – Partial bathing, called also stuping, which is applying hot flannels to any part of the body, dipped in medication decoctions whereby the steams breathe into the parts, and discuss obstructed humours.

Fundament – The back part of the lower body or buttocks.

Grains – A figure of measurement.

Gravel – In this instance, *gravel* refers to sandy matter concreted in the kidneys, or kidney stones.

Gripings – Pain in the bowels, or bellyache.

Herbal Simple – A single ingredient in a medicine; a drug, it is popularly used for a herb.

Herbal Simpling – To gather herbal simples.

Humor – The different kinds of moisture in the body, reckoned by the old physicians to be phlegm, blood, choler, and melancholy, which as the predominated, were supposed to determine the temper of mind.

Imposthumes – A collection of purulent matter in a bag or cyst.

Intermittents – Happening at intervals, usually referring to fever.

Isope – The middle English name for Hyssop.

Loaf Sugar – Sugar formed into the shape of a loaf.

Malific, Malefic(k) – Derived from the Latin term *Maleficium*: an act of witchcraft performed with the intention to cause harm or injury.

Materia Medica – Latin term for the history of pharmacy for the body, replaced in the modern world by the word pharmacology.

GLOSSARY

Megrim – Defined in modern medicine as similar to a migraine or severe headache.

Menses – Referring to menstruation or menstrual cycle.

Officinal – A herb, plant, drug, etc.: used in medicine or the arts.

Pappus – Crown of fruit of Compositae, and similar plants.

Perennial – Plants that live for two years or more.

Physic(k) – The art or practice of healing; the healing art; the medical profession. The medical faculty personified; physicians.

Physic Garden – A garden for the cultivation of medicinal plants.

Pleurisy – Inflammation of the pleura, with or without effusion of fluid into the pleural cavity; a disease characterised by pain in the chest or side, with fever or loss of appetite, etc.; usually caused by chill, or occurring as a complication of other diseases.

Pottle – A measure of capacity for liquids (also for corn and other dry goods, rarely for butter), equal to two quarts or half a gallon.

Poultice – A soft mass of some substance (as bread, meal, bran, linseed, various herbs, etc.), usually made with boiling water, and spread upon muslin, linen, or other material, applied to the skin to supply moisture or warmth, as an emollient for a sort or inflamed part.

Quart – The fourth part of a gallon.

Refrigerant – Cooling; mitigating heat.

Rheumatic – adj. of *Rheum*: Watery matter secreted by the mucous glands or membranes, such as collects in or drops from the nose, eyes, and mouth, etc., and which, when abnormal, was supposed to cause disease; hence, an excessive or morbid 'defluxion' of any kind. In this instance *Rheumatic* may refer to: Of persons, their bodies: suffering from a defluxion of rheum or catarrh.

Rubefacients – An application producing redness of the skin; esp. a counter irritant having this effect.

Stimulant – Something that temporarily quickens some vital process, or the function of some organ; a stimulant agent.

Stomachic – Of or pertaining to the stomach; gastric. Of an ailment: Caused by a disorder of the stomach. A stomachic medicine.

Suppuration – The process or condition of suppurating; the formation or secretion of pus; the coming to a head of a boil or other eruption.

Tincture – A solution, usually in a menstruum of alcohol, of some principle used in medicine, chiefly vegetable, as tincture of opium (*landanum*).

Tisane – Herbal infusion or tea made by steeping herbs and spices in hot water.

Tonic – Having the property of increasing or restoring the tone or healthy condition and activity of the system or organs; strengthening, invigorating, bracing (Of remedies or remedial treatment, and hence of air, climate, etc.). A tonic medicine, application or agent.

Tumour – A morbid swelling.

Uvula – Fleshy process hanging from the mouth palate at the back of the throat.

Verjuice – The acid juice of green or unripe grapes, crab apples, or other sour fruit, expressed and formed into a liquor; formerly much used in cooking, as a condiment, or for medicinal purposes.

Virtues – Qualities or traits of herbs, used in this instance to mostly describe medicinal properties.

Weal – The mark or ridge raised on the flesh by the blow of a rod, lash, etc.

Wyrd – An ancestral word to the modern English 'weird', leaning towards the more supernatural and uncanny.

HERB INDEX

BIBLIOGRAPHY

'Notes.' *Popular Science Monthly* III. 1873.

'The Woman's World'. *Mid Sussex Times*. 1895.

'Who'll Buy My Lavender.' *Napanee Express*. 18 February 1910.

Agar, Madeline. *Garden Design in Theory and Practice*. Philadelphia: J.B. Lippincott Company. 1912.

Agrippa, Cornelius von Nettesheim Heinrich. *The Philosophy of Natural Magic: A Complete Work on Natural Magic, White Magic, Black Magic*. Chicago: DeLaurence Co. 1913.

Anon. *Guide to Fortune-Telling by Dreams*. Boston: A. B. Courtney. 1894.

Anon. *The Famous Book of Herbs*. Bristol: King Press. 2013.

Anon. *Vaughan's Vegetable Cook Book: How to Cook and Use Rarer Vegetables and Herbs: A Boon to Housewives*. New York: Vaughan's Seed Store. 1919.

Arkell, Reginald. *Green Fingers – A Present for a Good Gardener*. Bristol: Gregg Press. 2011.

Aubrey, John. *Miscellanies upon Various Subjects*. London: Printed for W. Ottridge; and E. Easton, at Salisbury. 1784.

Bahia. *The Skilful Physician: Containing Directions for the Preservation of a Healthful Condition, and Approved Remedies for All Diseases and Infirmities (Outward or Inward) Incident to the Body of Man ... Whereunto Is Added Experimented Instructions for the Compounding of Perfumes, Also for the Chusing and Ordering of All Kinds of Wines, Both in Preserving the Sound, and Rectifying Those That Are Prick'd: Never Before Imparted to Publick View*. London: Printed by Tho. Maxey for Nath. Ekins. 1656.

Baring-Gould, Sabine, H. Fleetwood Sheppard, and F. W. Bussell. *Songs of the West; Folk Songs of Devon and Cornwall*. Boston: E.C. Schirmer Music Co. 1928.

Baring-Gould, Sabine. *An Old English Home: And Its Dependencies*. London: Methuen & Co. 1898.

Bean, W. J. *Hardy Ornamental Trees and Shrubs – With Chapters on Conifers, Sea-Side Planting and Trees for Towns*. Bristol: Camp Press. 2010.

Beeton, Isabella. *Gardening*. Bristol: Home Farm Books. 2016.

Bentley, Robert, and Henry Trimen. *Medicinal Plants. Being Descriptions With Original Figures of the Principal Plants Employed in Medicine and an Account of the Characters, Properties, and Uses of Their Parts and Products of Medicinal Value*. London: J. & A. Churchill. 1880.

Bickerdyke, John. *Curiosities of Ale and Beer*. London: Spring Books. 1889.

Biddle, Violet Purton. *Small Gardens, and How to Make the Most of Them*. London: C. Arthur Pearson Ltd. 1901.

Blackman, Winifred S. 'The Magical and Ceremonial Uses of Fire.' *Folklore 27*, no. 4,: 352–77. 1916.

Bowen, David. *Folklore Guide to the Weather*. Bristol: Read Country Books. 2018.

Brown, Oliver Phelps. *The Complete Herbalist: Or, the People Their Own Physicians, by the Use of Nature's Remedies ; Describing the Great Curative Properties Found in the Herbal Kingdom ; A New and Plain System of Hygienic Principles, Together With Comprehensive Essays on Sexual Philosophy, Marriage, Divorce*. London: Fredk W. Hale. 1885.

Burroughs, John. *Pepacton*. Boston and New York: Houghton, Mifflin and Co. 1881.

Burton, Robert. *The Anatomy of Melancholy: What It Is, With All the Kinds Causes, Symptomes, Prognostickes, & Seuerall Cures of It. In Three Partitions, With Their Seuerall Sections, Members & Subsections, Philosophically, Medicinally, Historically, Opened & Cut Up*. London: Crips & Lodo Lloyd. 1652.

Cameron, L. C. R. *The Wild Foods of Great Britain – Where to Find Them and How to Cook Them*. London: G. Routledge & Sons Ltd. 1917.

Cato, Marcus Porcius, and Heinrich Keil. *De Agri Cultura*. Lipsiae: Teubner. 1894.

Chambers, Robert. *The Popular Rhymes of Scotland, with Illustrations, Chiefly Collected from Oral Sources*. Edinburgh: William Hunter. 1826.

Child, Lydia Maria. *The American Frugal Housewife*. Massachusetts: Applewood Books. 1829.

Cielo, Astra. *Signs, Omens and Superstitions*. New York: G. Sully & Company. 1918.

Clare, John. *Poems by John Clare*. Rugby: The Rugby Press. 1901.

Clare, John. *The Shepherd's calendar with village stories, and other poems*. London: Taylor. 1827.

BIBLIOGRAPHY

Clare, John. *The Village Minstrel, and Other Poems*. London: Taylor and Hessey. 1821.

Cobbett, Anne. *The English Housekeeper, or, Manual of Domestic Management*. Sixthed. London: A. Cobbett. 1851.

Coles, William. *Adam in Eden; Or, Natures Paradise. The History of Plants, Fruits, Herbs and Flowers. With Their Several Names, Whether Greek, Latin or English.*. London: Printed by J. Streater, for Nathaniel Brooke. 1657.

Columella, Lucius Junius Moderatus. *L. Junius Moderatus Columella of Husbandry. In Twelve Books. And His Book Concerning Trees*. London: Printed for A. Millar. 1745.

Cowper, William. *The Works of William Cowper – Comprising of His Poems, Correspondence, and Translations*. Edited by Robert South. VI. Vol. VI. London: H. G. Bohn. 1854.

Coxe, John Redman, and Joseph Fox. *The Philadelphia Medical Dictionary: Containing a Concise Explanation of All the Terms Used in Medicine, Surgery, Pharmacy. Botany, Natural History, Chymistry, and Materia Medica. Compiled From the Best Authorities...* Philadelphia: Thomas and George Palmer. 1808.

Culpeper, Nicholas. *Complete Herbal, to Which Is Now Added Upwards of One Hundred Additional Herbs, with a Display of Their Medicinal and Occult Qualities: Physically Applied to the Cure of All Disorders Incident to Mankind*. London: Kelly. 1824.

Curtis, Mary Isabel. *Stories in Trees*. Chicago: Lyons & Carnahan. 1925.

Dadant, Camille Pierre. *Facts About Honey – What Honey Is, How It Is Taken from the Bees, Its Value as Food and Honey Recipes*. 1916.

Dover Wilson, John. *Life in Shakespeare's England: A Book of Elizabethan Prose*. Bristol: Hesperides Press. 2008.

Drayton, Michael. *Minor Poems of Michael Drayton*. Edited by Cyril Brett. Oxford: Clarendon Press. 1907.

Drayton, Michael. *The Complete Works of Michael Drayton – Polyolbion, and the Harmony of the Church*. London: Smith. 1876.

Dunglison, Robley. *General Therapeutics and Materia Medica: Adapted for a Medical Text Book*. Philadelphia: Lea and Blanchard. 1850.

Earle, Alice Morse. *Old-Time Gardens; Newly Set Forth, a Book of the Sweet O' the Year*. Norwood: Macmillan. 1901.

Eaton, Mary. *The Cook and Housekeeper's Complete and Universal Dictionary: Including a System of Modern Cookery in All Its Various Branches, Adapted to the Use of Private Families: Also a Variety of Original and Valuable Information Relative to Baking, Brewing, Carving ... And Every Other Subject Connected With Domestic Economy*. Bungay: J. & R. Childs. 1822.

Ecclesiasticus 38:4 King James Bible.

Ellacombe, Henry N. *Plant-Lore & Garden-Craft of Shakespeare*. London: W. Satchell and Co. 1884.

Ellet, Elizabeth F. *The Women of the American Revolution*. New York: Baker and Scribner. 1849.

Ellis, David. *Medicinal Herbs and Poisonous Plants*. London: Blackie and Son. 1918.

Evelyn, John. *Acetaria*. London: Tooke. 1699.

Every Woman's Encyclopaedia. Vol. II. 1800.

Fernie, William Thomas. *Herbal Simples: Approved for Modern Uses of Cure*. Bristol: John Wright & Co. 1897.

Fludd, Robert. *Utriusque Cosmi maioris scilicet et minoris metaphysica, physica atque Technica Historia: In duo Volumnina Secundum cosmi Differentiam Diuisa*. Oppenhemii: Aere Johan-Theodori de Bry, typis Hieronymi Galleri. 1617.

Folkard, Richard. *Plant Lore, Legends, and Lyrics, Embracing the Myths, Traditions, Superstitions, and Folk-Lore of the Plant Kingdom*. London: S. Low. 1884.

Foster, Frank Pierce. *Reference-Book of Practical Therapeutics*. New York: D. Appleton & Company. 1897.

Frazer, James George. *The Golden Bough: A Study in Comparative Religion*. London: Macmillan and Co. 1894.

Gerard, John. *The Herball, or Generall Historie of Plantes*. London: Printed by A. Islip, J. Norton and R. Whitakers. 1636.

Gibson, Wilfrid Wilson. *Battle*. London: Mathews. 1915.

Gomme, George Laurence. *Folklore as an Historical Science*. London: Meuthen & Co. 1908.

Gordon, Elizabeth. *Mother Earth's Children: The Frolics of Fruit and Vegetables*. New York: Wise-Parslow Co. 1914.

Goudiss, C. Houston, and Alberta M. Goudiss. *Foods That Will Win the War, and How to Cook Them*. New York: Forecast Pub. Co. 1918.

Gregory, Augusta. *Visions and Beliefs in the West of Ireland*. New York: G.P. Putnam's Sons. 1920.

Grieve, Maude. *A modern herbal : the medicinal, culinary, cosmetic and economic properties, cultivation and folklore of herbs, grasses, fungi, shrubs and trees with all their modern scientific uses*. New York: Dover. 1931.

Grieve, Maude. *Culinary Herbs: How to Grow and Where to Sell; With an Account of Their Uses and History; Specially Written to Assist Members of the British Guild of Herb Growers*. British Guild of Herb Growers. 1890.

Hall, Joseph, and Josiah Pratt. *The Works of Joseph Hall: Now First Collected, With Some Account of His Life and Sufferings*. London: C. Whittingham for Williams and Smith. 1808.

Harder, Jules Arthur. *The Physiology of Taste; Harder's Book of Practical American Cookery (In Six Volumes), Vol. I*. San Francisco. 1885.

Harland, John, and T. T. Wilkinson. *Lancashire Folk-Lore: Illustrative of the Superstitious Beliefs and Practices, Local Customs and Usages of the People of the County Palatine*. London: John Heywood. 1882.

Hawthorne, Diana. *Laurie's Complete Fortune Teller*. London: W. & G. Foyle. 1946.

Herman Senn, Charles. *A pocket dictionary of foods & culinary encyclopaedia*. London: Food and Cookery Publishing Company. 1908.

Housman, A. E. *Last Poems: With a Chapter from Twenty-Four Portraits*. Bristol: Yoakum Press. 2020.

Howes, Frank N. *Plants and Beekeeping*. Faber & Faber. 1945.

Hudson, William Henry. *Far Away and Long Ago*. London: J. M. Dent & Sons. 1918.

Jerrold, Tom. *Our War-Time Kitchen Garden: The Plants We Grow and How We Cook Them*. London: Chatto & Windus. 1917.

Johnson, Samuel. *A Dictionary of the English Language: In Which the Words Are Deduced From Their Originals, and Illustrated in Their Different Significations by Examples From the Best Writers: To Which Are Prefixed a History of the Language, and an English Grammar*. Vols. I & II. London. 1755.

Juno, Madame. *The Gypsy Queen Dream Book and Fortune Teller*. London: Herbert Jenkins. 1930.

Kains, Maurice Grenville. *Culinary Herbs: Their Cultivation, Harvesting, Curing, and Uses*. New York: Orange Judd Company. 1912.

Keats, John. *The Poetical Works of John Keats*. London: Reeves & Turner. 1895.

Keats, John. *The Works of John Keats*. Bristol: Becker Press. 2008.

Kipling, Rudyard. *Best of Rudyard Kipling – A Collection of Essential Poetry*. Bristol: Ragged Hand. 2020.

Kittredge, George Lyman. *The Old Farmer and His Almanack – Being Some Observations on Life and Manners in New England a Hundred Years Ago Suggested by Reading the Earlier Numbers of Mr. Robert B. Thomas's Farmer's Almanack, Together With Extracts Curious, Instructive and Entertaining as Well as a Variety of Miscellaneous Matter*. Cambridge: Harvard University Press. 1920.

Klickmann, Flora. *The Flower-Patch Among the Hills*. 1918

Leigh, Hunt James Henry, and Herbert Railton. *Poems of Leigh Hunt: With Prefaces from Some of His Periodicals*. London: J. M. Dent & Co. 1891.

Leland, Charles Godfrey. *Gypsy Sorcery and Fortune Telling*. New York: Charles Scribner's Sons. 1891.

Leyel, Hilda. *Herbal Delights: Tisanes, Syrups, Confections, Electuaries, Robs, Juleps, Vinegars and Conserves*. London: Faber. 1937.

Longfellow, Henry Wadsworth. *Ballads and Other Poems*. Cambridge: John Owen. 1842.

Longfellow, Henry Wadsworth. *The Complete Poetical Works of Henry Wadsworth Longfellow: Cambridge Edition*. Boston: Houghton Mifflin and Company. 1851.

Lowell, James Russell. *Poems of James Russell Lowell*. New York: Thomas Y. Crowell & Co. 1892.

Lyndoe, Edward. *Everybody's Book of Fate and Fortune*. London: Odhams Press. 1937.

MacAlister, Charles J. *Comfrey – An Ancient Medicinal Remedy*. Bristol: Lowrie Press. 2012.

Madinger Willich, Anthony Florian. *Domestic Encyclopedia*. London: Murray and Highley. 1802.

Mare, Walter de la. *The Sunken Garden, and Other Poems*. London: Beaumont Press. 1917.

Mathers, S. Liddell Macgregor. *The Key of Solomon the King*. London: George Redway. 1889.

McKay, C. D. *The French Garden: A Diary and Manual of Intensive Cultivation*. London: Associated Newspapers. 1908.

Millay, Edna St. Vincent. *Afternoon on a Hill – Love Letters to Nature*. Bristol: Ragged Hand. 2020.

Millay, Edna St. Vincent. *Second April – The Poetry of Edna St. Vincent Millay; with a Biography by Carl Van Doren*. Bristol: Ragged Hand. 2020.

BIBLIOGRAPHY

Milton, John. *Milton's Paradise Lost*. Edited by D.C. Somervell. London: J. M. Dent & Sons. 1920.

Montgomery Skinner, Charles. *Myths and Legends of Flowers, Fruits and Plants*. Philadelphia: J. B. Lippincott Co. 1911.

Morton, John William. *250 Beautiful Flowers and How to Grow Them*. Bristol: Home Farm Books. 2009.

Murray, James A. H., and Henry Bradley. *A New English Dictionary on Historical Principles: Founded Mainly on the Materials Collected by the Philological Society*. Oxford: Clarendon Press. 1897.

Murray, James A. H., Henry Bradley, William A. Craigie, and C. T. Onions. *The Oxford English Dictionary: Being A Corrected Re-issue with an Introduction, Supplement, and Bibliography of A New English Dictionary on Historical Principles Founded Mainly on the Materials Collected by the Philogical Society*. 11 vols. Oxford: Clarendon Press, 1933.

Neil, Marion Harris. *Canning, Preserving and Pickling*. London: W. & R. Chambers. 1914.

Northcote, Lady Rosalind. *The Book of Herbs*. London: The Bodley Head. 1903.

Ovid. *Ovids Metamorphosis: Englished, Mythologiz'd, and Represented in Figures: An Essay to the Translation of Virgil's Æneis*. Translated by George Sandys. London: J. L. for Andrew Hebb. 1640.

Parkinson, John, and Thomas Cotes. *Theatrum Botanicum: The Theater of Plants: Or, an Herball of Large Extent: Containing Therein a More Ample and Exact History and Declaration of the Physicall Herbs and Plants... Distributed Into Sundry Classes or Tribes, for the More Easie Knowledge of the Many Herbes of One Nature and Property...* London: Tho. Cotes. 1640.

Paxton, Joseph, and Samuel Hereman. *Paxton's Botanical Dictionary; Comprising the Names, History, and Culture of All Plants Known in Britain; With a Full Explanation of Technical Terms. New Ed. Including All the New Plants up to the Present Year*. London: Bradbury, Evans, & Co. 1868.

Petulengro, Gipsy. *A Romany Life: With 4 Illustrations*. London: Methuen & Co. 1935.

Petulengro, Gipsy. *Romany Remedies and Recipes*. London: Methuen & Co. 1935.

Plat, Hugh. *Delights for Ladies: To Adorn Their Persons, Tables, Closet's and Distillatories: With Beauties, Banquets, Perfumes and Waters*. London: James Young. 1644.

Pliny, Elder. *The Natural History of Pliny*. Translated by John Bostock. Vol. IV. London: Bohn. 1857.

Porta, Giambattista della. *Natural Magick by John Baptista Porta, a Neapolitane: In Twenty Books: Wherein Are Set Forth All the Riches and Delights of the Natural Sciences*. London: Printed for Thomas Young, and Samuel Speed. 1658.

Porteous, Alexander. *Forest Folklore, Mythology and Romance*. London: Allen & Unwin. 1928.

Proust, Marcel. *Swann's Way: Remembrance of Things Past*. I. Vol. I. New York: Henry Holt and Company. 1922.

Quelch, Mary Thorne. *The Herb Garden*. London: Faber. 1951.

Quiller-Couch, Arthur. *The Oxford Book of English Verse 1250 – 1900*. Oxford: Claredon Press. 1926.

Radford, Edwin, and Mona Augusta Radford. *Encyclopaedia of Superstitions*. Bristol: Pierides Press. 2008.

Ravenscroft, Thomas. *Deuteromelia: Or, the Second Part of Musicks Melodie, or Melodius Musicke of Pleasant Roundelaies ; K.H. Mirth, or Freemen's Songs and Such Delightfull Catches. by T.R., I.e. Thomas Ravenscroft*. London: For T. Adams. 1609.

Read, Carveth. *The Origin of Man and of His Superstitions*. London: Cambridge University Press. 1920.

Richards, Gertrude Moore. *The Melody of Earth; An Anthology of Garden and Nature Poems From Present-Day Poets*. Boston: Houghton Mifflin Company. 1918.

Rickett, F. C. *Rollright Stones: History and Legends in Prose and Poetry – With Five Illustrations*. Chipping Norton: Percy Simms & Son. 1900.

Ripley, George, Charles A. Dana, William Augustus Leggo, and Henry Draper. *The American Cyclopaedia: A Popular Dictionary of General Knowledge*. New York: D. Appleton and Co. 1881.

Robinson, Clement, and Edward Arber. *A Handful of Pleasant Delights. Containing Sundry New Sonnets and Delectable Histories in Divers Kinds of Metre...* London. 1878.

Robinson, Mary. *Sappho and Phaon: In a Series of Legitimate Sonnets, with Thoughts on Poetical Subjects, Etc.* London: S. Gosnell. 1796.

Robinson, Matthew. *The New Family Herbal: Comprising a Description, and the Medical Virtues of British and Foreign Plants, Founded on the Works of Eminent Modern English and American Writers on the Medical Properties of Herbs: To Which Is Added, the Botanic Family Physician; Valuable Medical Receipts; And Important Directions Regarding Diet, Clothing, Bathing, Air, Exercise, &C., &C.* London: William Nicholson & Sons. 1863.

BIBLIOGRAPHY

Rohde, Eleanour Sinclair. 'The Making of the Bee Garden'. *The Times*. 1939

Rohde, Eleanour Sinclair. *A Garden of Herbs*. London: The Medici Society. 1921.

Rohde, Eleanour Sinclair. *Herbs and Herb Gardening*. London: Medici Society. 1936.

Rohde, Eleanour Sinclair. *The Old English Herbals*. London: Longmans. 1922.

Rohde, Eleanour Sinclair. *The Scented Garden*. London: The Medici Society. 1900.

Rundell, Maria Eliza Ketelby. *A New System of Domestic Cookery Formed Upon Principles of Economy, and Adapted to the Use of Private Families: With the Addition of Many New Receipts, and Embellished With Engravings*. Halifax: Milner and Sowerby. 1866.

Rutherfurd Ely, Helena. *The Practical Flower Garden*. London: The Macmillan Company. 1913.

Scott, Mary Augusta. Ed. *The Essays of Francis Bacon*. New York, Chicago, Boston: Charles Scribner's Sons. 1908.

Senn, Charles Herman. *Senn's Culinary Encyclopaedia; a Dictionary of Technical Terms, the Names of All Foods, Food and Cookery Auxiliaries, Condiments and Beverages, Specially Adapted for Use by Chefs, Hotel and Restaurant Managers, Cookery Teachers, Housekeepers, Etc.*. London: Spottiswoode & Co. 1898.

Seymour, John D. *Irish Witchcraft and Demonology*. Baltimore: Norman, Remington. 1913.

Shakespeare, William. *Hamlet*. Bristol: Read & Co. Classics. 2010.

Shakespeare, William. *Othello*. Bristol: Read & Co. Classics. 2010.

Shakespeare, William. *Romeo and Juliet*. Bristol: Read & Co. Classics. 2010.

Shakespeare, William. *The Winter's Tale*. Bristol: Read & Co. Classics. 2011.

Shelley, Percy Bysshe. *The Complete Poetical Works of Percy Bysshe Shelley. Edited by Thomas Hutchinson*. London: Gibbings and Company, Limited. 1914.

Sigourney, Lydia Huntley. *Pocahontas and Other Poems*. New York: Harper and Brothers. 1841.

Sikes, Wirt. *Quaint Old Customs of Wales (Folklore History Series)*. Bristol: Pierides Press. 2016.

Simmonite, William Joseph, A. M. & Nicholas Culpeper. *The Herbal Remedies of Culpeper and Simmonite – Nature's Medicine*. London: W. Foulsham & Co. 1957.

Singleton, Esther. *The Shakespeare Garden: With Numerous Illustrations From Photographs And Reproductions Of Old Wood Cuts*. New York: Century Co. 1922.

Spenser, Edmund. The Faerie Queene. *Disposed into Twelve Bookes, Fashioning XII*. London: Printed for William Ponsonbie. 1596.

Spratt, G. *Flora Medica: Containing Coloured Delineations of the Various Medicinal Plants Admitted Into the London, Edinburgh and Dublin Pharmacopoeias, With Their Natural History, Botanical Descriptions, Medical and Chemical Properties, Etc. ; Together With a Concise Introduction to Botany, a Copious Glossary of Botanical Terms and a List of Poisonous Plants, Etc*. London: Callow & Wilson. 1829.

Stillé, Alfred, and John M. Maisch. *The National Dispensatory: Containing the Natural History, Chemistry, Pharmacy, Actions and Uses of Medicines, Including Those Recognized in the Pharmacopoeias of the United States and Great Britain*. Philadelphia: Henry C. Lea. 1879.

Stoker, Bram. *Dracula*. Bristol: Fantasy and Horror Classics. 2019.

T., A., and George Wateson. *A Rich Storehouse or Treasurie for the Diseased.: Wherein Are Many Approved Medicines for Divers and Sundry Diseases, Which Have Beene Long Hidden and Not Come to Light Before This Time. First Set Foorth for the Benefit and Comfort of the Poorer Sort of People, That Are Not of Ability to Goe to the Phisitions*. London: Thomas Purfoot & Ralph Blower. 1616.

Taunt, Henry. *The Rollright Stones; the Stonehenge of Oxfordshire: With Some Account of the Ancient Druids, and Sagas Rendered Into English*. Oxford: H. W. Taunt & Co. 1907.

Tennyson, Alfred Lord. The Works Of Alfred Lord Tennyson. London: Macmillan and Co. 1893.

The A–Z of Caramels. Bristol: Two Magpies Publishing. 2014.

The A–Z of Homemade Chutneys, Pickles, and Relishes. Bristol: Two Magpies Publishing. 2014.

The A–Z of Homemade Jams and Jellies. Bristol: Two Magpies Publishing. 2014.

The A–Z of Homemade Syrups and Cordials. Bristol: Two Magpies Publishing. 2014.

Thiselton Dyer, Thomas Firminger. 'Plants in Witchcraft.' *Popular Science Monthly*. April 1889.

Thistelton-Dyer, Thomas Firminger. *The Folk-Lore of Plants*. Piccadilly: Chatto & Windus. 1889.

BIBLIOGRAPHY

Thomas, H. H. *Pruning Made Easy – How to Prune Rose Trees, Fruit Trees and Ornamental Trees and Shrubs*. London: Cassell & Company. 1927.

Thomson, Anthony Todd. *The London Dispensatory*. London: Longman. 1811.

Thorpe, Benjamin. *Northern Mythology: Comprising the Principal Popular Traditions and Superstitions of Scandinavia, North Germany, and the Netherlands*. Miami: Hardpress. 1851.

Topsell, Edward. *The History of Four-Footed Beasts and Serpents: Describing at Large Their True and Lively Figure, Their Several Names, Conditions, Kinds, Virtues (Both Natural and Medicinal), Countries of Their Breed, Their Love and Hatred to Mankind, and the Wonderful Work of God in Their Creation, Preservation, and Destruction: Interwoven With Curious Variety of Historical Narrations Out of Scriptures, Fathers, Philosophers, Physicians, and Poets: Illustrated With Divers Hieroglyphicks and Emblems, &C. Both Pleasant and Profitable for Students in All Faculties and Professions*. London: Printed by E. Cotes, for G. Sawbridge. 1658.

Turner, Robert, and Obadiah Blagrave. *Botanologia. the British Physician: Or, the Nature and Vertues of English Plants: Exactly Describing Such Plants as Grow Naturally in Our Land with Their Several Names, Greek, Latine, or English Natures, Places Where They Grow, Times When They Flourish, and Are Most Proper to Be Gathered ; Their Degrees of Temperature, Applications Andvertues, Physical and Astrological Uses, Treated of ; Each Plant Appropriated to the Several Diseases They Cure and Directions for Their Medicinal Uses, throughout the Whole Body of Man ..* London: Obadiah Blagrave. 1687.

Tusser, Thomas, and William Fordyce Mavor. *Five Hundred Points of Good Husbandry, as Well for the Champion or Open Country, as for the Woodland or Several; Together With a Book of Huswifery. Being a Calendar of Rural and Domestic Economy, for Every Month in the Year; And Exhibiting a Picture of the Agriculture, Customs, and Manners of England, in the Sixteenth Century*. London: Lackington, Allen, and Co. 1812.

Tuxford, Hester H. *Miss Tuxford's Modern Cookery for the Middle Classes: Hints on Modern Gas Stove Cooking*. Tattershall: Simpkin, Marshall Ltd.; John Heywood Ltd. 1933.

Various. *Gleanings from Gloucestershire Housewives – Traditional Recipes*. Gloucester: Gloucestershire Federation of Women's Institutes. 1936.

Various. *Secrets of Some Wiltshire Housewives: A Book of Recipes – Collected from the Members of Women's Institutes*. Coates & Parker: Warminster. 1927.

Warner Morley, Margaret. *Honey-Makers*. Chicago: A.C. McClurg and Company. 1899.

White, Florence. *Good Things in England: A Practical Cookery Book for Everyday Use, Containing Traditional and Regional Recipes Suited to Modern Tastes*. London, Toronto, New York: Jonathan Cape. 1932.

Whitman, Walt. *Leaves of Grass*. Bristol: Pomona Press. 2008.

Wilde, Jane. *Ancient Legends, Mystic Charms and Superstitions of Ireland: With Sketches of the Irish Past*. London: Chattoo. 1919.

Williams, Ralp. *A Black Almanack or Predictions and Astronimonicall Observations Foreshewing What Will Happen to the King of Scots This Present Year, From the Aspect and Conjunction of the Planets on the Day and Hour of His Coronation the First of January 1651. Also Some Calculations Concerning Many Bloudy Fights Between the English and Scots and the Various Success Thereof. With a Bloudy Contention Between the Buff-Coat, the Long Coat, and the Black-Coat, and the Issne [Sic] Thereof. Licensed According to Order*. London: Printed by J. Clowes. 1651.

Willich, Anthony Florian Madinger. *The Domestic Encyclopaedia*. IV. Vol. IV. London: Murray & Highle. 1802.

Wood, John. *Hardy Perennials and Old-Fashioned Garden Flowers: Describing the Most Desirable Plants for Borders, Rockeries, and Shrubberies, Including Foliage as Well as Flowering Plants*. London: L. Upcott Gill. 1884.

Woodward, Marcus. *How to Enjoy Flowers: The New Flora Historica*. London: Hodder and Stoughton. 1928.

Woodward, Marcus. *Mistress of Stantons Farm*. Heath Cranton Limited. 1938.

Woodward, William Arthur, and Marcus Woodward. *The Countryman's Jewel; Days in the Life of a Sixteenth Century Squire*. London: Chapman & Hall. 1934.

Wright, Walter P. *The Perfect Garden, How to Keep It Beautiful and Fruitful: With Practical Hints on Economical Management and the Culture of All the Principal Flowers, Fruits, and Vegetables: Illustrated With Coloured Plates, Engravings, and Plans*. London: Grant Richards. 1909.

BIBLIOGRAPHY OF ILLUSTRATIONS

Abbildungen Aller Medizinisch-öKonomisch-Technologischen Gewächse. Vienna. 1818. 216

Anazarbos, Dioscorides Pedanius, of. *De materia medica by Pedanios Dioscorides of Anazarbos (fl. 1st century A.D.) translated into Arabic from the Syriac translation of Hunayn ibn Isḥāq al-'Ibādī (809?-873) by Mihrân ibn Mansûr ibn Mîhrân (fl. 12th cent.).* Tehran. 1889–1890. .... 42, 159

Argenta, Vicente Martin de. *Album de la Flora Médico-Farmacéutica é Industrial, Indígena y Exótica.* Madrid. 1862–1864......... 136

Baxter, William. *British Phænogamous Botany, or, Figures and Descriptions of the Genera of British Flowering Plants.* Oxford. 1834–1843. .... 6, 66–67, 106–107, 165

Bertuch, Friedrich and Carl. *Picture-Book for Children: Containing a Pleasant Collection of Animals, Plants, Fruits, Minerals.* Weimar. 1795... 221

Bonelli, Giorgio. *Hortus Romanus Juxta Systems Tournefortianum Paulo. Sumptibus Bouchard et Gravier.* 1772–1793. ...... 4, 19, 38, 45, 140–141, 192–193, 198

Bulliard, Pierre. *Flora Parisiensis, ou, Descriptions ET Figures Des Plantes Qui Croissent Aux Environs de Paris.* Paris: P. F. Didot. 1776–1783. 60

Catto, William. *Common Stinging Nettle.* Aberdeen: Scotland. 1915.. 166

Collection, Wellcome. *Roots of Ginger (Zingiber Officinale) And of Dropwort (Filipendula Vulgaris).* Watercolour. 118

Crane, Walter. *Flowers From Shakespeare's Garden: A Posy From the Plays.* London: Cassell & Co. 1909. 135

Curtis, William. *Flora Londinensis, or, Plates and Descriptions of Such Plants as Grow Wild in the Environs of London.* London: B. White. 1777. 82

Duthie, John Firminger. *Field and Garden Crops of the North-Western Provinces and Oudh.* Roorkee: Thomason Civil Engineering College Press. 1882–1893... 112

Eisenberger, Nicolaus Friedrich. *Herbarium Blackwellianum Emendatum et Auctum, ID EST, Elisabethae Blackwell Collectio Stirpium.* Norimbergae. 1750–1754.. 54–55, 173, 197

Flora and Thalia; Or, Gems of Flowers and Poetry: Being an Alphabetical Arrangement of Flowers, With Appropriate Poetical Illustrations, Embellished With Coloured Plates. Philadelphia: Carey, Lea, and Blanchard. 1836. 132

Fludd, Robert. *'Integrae Naturae Speculum Artisque Imago' – The Mirror of the Whole of Nature and the Image of Art, Utriusque Cosmi Maioris Scilicet ET Minoris Metaphysica, Physica Atque Technica Historia.* Oppenhemii. 1617................... 35

Garsault, François Alexandre de. *Les Figures Des Plantes et Animaux D'Usage en Medecine, Décrits Dans la Matiere Medicale de Geoffroy Medecin.* Paris: Desprez. 1764–1765. 133

George Spratt. *Flora Medica.* London: Callow and Wilson. 1829........................... 52, 110, 142, 208, 244

Gordon, Elizabeth. *Mother Earth's Children, the Frolics of Fruits and Vegetables.* New York: The Wise-Parslow Company. 1914..... 177

Hall, Charles Albert. *Plant-Life.* London: A. & C. Black. 1915... 72

Haller, Albrecht von. *Alberti Halleri D. de Allii Genere Naturali Libellus.* Gottingae: Typis A. Vandenhoeck. 1745............ 111

Hamilton, Edward. *Novæ Hollandiæ Plantarum Specimenthe Flora Homoeopathica: Or, Illustrations and Descriptions of the Medicinal Plants Used as Homoeopathic Remedies.* London: Leath & Ross. 1853. .... 96, 194, 234–235

Hamilton, Edward. *The Flora Homoeopathica: Or, Illustrations and Descriptions of the Medicinal Plants Used as Homoeopathic Remedies.* London, Leath & Ros. 1852... 154

Hibberd, Shirley. *Familiar Garden Flowers.* London: Cassell. 1907.. 39

Hoppe, David Heinrich. *Ectypa Plantarum Ratisbonensium.* Regensburg. 1789–1790. 90

Hulme, F. Edward. *Familiar Wild Flowers Figured and Described.* London: Cassell and Company. 1878................. 11, 16

Johns, Charles Alexander. *Flowers of the Field.* London: Society for Promoting Christian Knowledge. 1911. .... 105, 213, 243

Kniphof, Johann Hieronymus. *Atlas de Poche Des Plantes Des Champs, Des Prairies ET Des Bois: A L'Usage Des Promeneurs ET Des Excursionnistesd.* Halae Magdeburgicae: MDCCLVIII-MDCCLXIV. 1758.. 18

Köhler, Hermann Adolph. *Köhler's Medizinal-Pflanzen in Naturgetreuen Abbildungen MIT Kurz Erläuterndem Texte – Volume II.* Gera-Untermhaus, Fr. Eugen Köhler. 1883.......... 3, 23, 50, 80, 93, 94, 128, 153, 170, 179, 193, 200, 228, 237

BIBLIOGRAPHY OF ILLUSTRATIONS

Kompagnie., *Lukas Hochenleitter UND. Plantarum Indigenarum ET Exoticarum Icones Ad Vivum Coloratae, Oder, Sammlung Nach Der Natur Gemalter Abbildungen Inn- UND Ausländlicher Pflanzen, Für Liebhaber UND Beflissene Der Botanik*. 1779. . . . . 79, 99

Labillardière, Jacques Julien Houton de. *Novæ Hollandiæ Plantarum Specimen*. Paris. 1804–1806. 90

Ledebour, Carl Friedrich von. *Icones Plantarum Novarum Vel Imperfecte Cognitarum Floram Rossicam, Imprimis Altaicam, Illustrantes*. Rigae: I. Deubner. 1829–1830. 83

Lyman, Henry Munson. *The Book of Health*. Rhode Island: W. P. Mason. 1898. 113

Mann, Johann Gottlieb. *Deutschlands Wildwachsende Arzney-Pflanzen*. Stuttgart: Zu haben bei dem Herausgeber. 1828. 201

Marble, Charles C. *Birds and All Nature*. Chicago: Nature Study Publishing Co. 1899. 119

Mather, S. Liddell MacGregor. *The Key of Solomon the King*. London: George Redway. 1889. 20

Mentz, August. *Billeder AF Nordens Flora*. København, G. E. C. Gad's Forlag. 1917–1927. . . . . 12, 232

Miller, Joseph. *A Curious Herbal - Containing Five Hundred Cuts, of the Most Useful Plants, Which Are Now Used in the Practice of Physick Engraved on Folio Copper Plates, After Drawings Taken From the Life By Elizabeth Blackwell. To Which Is Added a Short Description of Ye Plants and Their Common Uses in Physick*. London: Printed for Samuel Harding. 1737. . . 8, 14, 20, 26, 31, 46–47, 76, 86, 101, 133, 139, 150-151, 156, 162, 172, 186, 204, 218, 226–227

Millspaugh, Charles Frederick. *American Medicinal Plants; An Illustrated and Descriptive Guide to the American Plants Used as Homopathic Remedies: Their History, Preparation, Chemistry and Physiological Effects*. New York: Boericke & Tafel. c. 1887. . . . . . 69, 182

Monceau, M. Duhamel du. *Traité Des Arbres et Arbustes Que L'on Cultive en France en Pleine Terre*. Paris. 1801–1819. . . . . . . 13, 27, 51, 129, 189, 225

Moninckx, Jan & Maria. *Moninckx Atlas: Catalog in the Form of a Painted Herbarium of the Plants in the Hortus Medicus of the City of Amsterdam*. Amsterdam. c. 1699–1706. 198

Morss, John Stephenson and James. *Medical Botany*. London Printed for J. Churchill. 1836. 21

Munting, Abraham. *Phytographia Curiosa: Acetosa Vulgaris Sive Rumex Canpferinus*. Netherlands. c. 1700. 36

Nicholas Culpeper,. *Culpepper's Complete Herbal*. London: Richard Evans. 1815. 211

Oldberg, Oscar. *A Companion to the United States Pharmacopia*. New York: W. Wood & Co. 1884. 115

Otto Carl Berg. *Atlas Der Officinellen Pflanzen: Darstellung UND Beschreibung Der Im Arzneibuche Für Das Deutsche Reich Erwähnten Gewächse*. Leipzig: A. Felix. 1891. . . . . 84, 184, 190–191, 205, 229

Parsons, Frances Theodora. *How to Know the Wild Flowers: A Guide to the Names, Haunts and Habits of Our Common Wild Flowers*. New York: Scribner's. 1893. 181

Penzig, Ottone. *Flore Coloriée de Poche du Littoral Méditerranéen de Gênes à Barcelone Y Compris la Corse*. Paris, P. Klincksieck. 1902. 29

Rohde, Eleanour Sinclair. *The Making of the Bee Garden*. The Times. 1939. 23

Roscoe, William. *Monandrian Plants of the Order Scitamineae: Chiefly Drawn From Living Specimens in the Botanic Garden at Liverpool, Arranged According to the System of Linnaeus With Descriptions and Observations*. Liverpool: George Smith. 1828. 116

Rossi, Domenico de. *Raccolta Di Statue Antiche E Moderne*. Roma: Nella Stamperia alla Pace. 1704. 57

Scheidl, Franz Anton von. *Basil (Ocimum Basilicum L.): Entire Flowering Plant With Separate Floral Segments*. Vienna: Leopold Johann Kaliwoda. 1776. 43

Schmeil, Otto. *Lehrbuch Der Botanik; Für Höhere Lehranstalten UND Die Hand des Lehrers, Sowie Für Alle Freunde Der Natur. Unter Besonderer Berücksichtigung Biologischer Verhältnisse Bearb. von Otto Schmeil*. Leipzig: Quelle & Meyer. 1911. 32

Schmeil, Otto. *Pflanzen Der Heimat. Eine Auswahl Der Verbreitetsten Pflanzen Unserer Fluren in Wort und Bild*. Leipzig: Quelle und Meyer. 1913. . . . . 164, 212–213

Senn, Gustav. *Alpen-Flora : Westalpen*. Heidelberg: C. Winter. 1906. 131

Siélain, R. *Atlas de Poche Des Plantes Des Champs, Des Prairies et Des Bois: A L'Usage Des Promeneurs ET Des Excursionnistes*. Paris, P. Klincksieck. 1895. . . . . 17, 22, 68, 85, 104, 233

Sowerby, James. *English Botany, or, Coloured Figures of British Plants*. London: R. Hardwicke. 1865. 176–177

Step, Edward. *Favourite Flowers of Garden and Greenhouse*. London and New York: Frederick Warne & Co. 1897. 148

BIBLIOGRAPHY OF ILLUSTRATIONS

Step, Edward. *Wayside and Woodland Blossoms: A Pocket Guide to British Wild-Flowers for the Country Rambler.* London, F. Warne. 1895..63, 169

Stephenson, John. *Medical Botany.* 1836. ....88, 114, 134, 185, 196

Sturm, Jakob. *Deutschlands Flora in Abbildungen Nach Der Natur, Nurnberg. Gedruckt Auf Kosten Des Verfassers.* 1800.........9, 30, 34, 150, 241

Sturm, Jakob. *Sturms Flora von Deutschland.* Stuttgart: K. G. Lutz. 1900–1906. 217

Thomé, Otto Wilhelm. *Prof. Dr Thomé's Flora of Germany, Austria and Switzerland, in Words and Pictures, for School and Home.* Gera. 1889. ....7, 24, 37, 66–67, 86, 126, 130, 152–153, 168, 230, 240

Various. *Curtis's Botanical Magazine.* London: Academic Press. 1879..70

Various. *Curtis's Botanical Magazine.* London: Academic Press. 1907...102

Various. *Flore Médicale.* Paris, Imprimerie de C. L. F. Panckoucke. 1834..............10, 28, 40, 53, 64, 78, 98, 122, 175, 181, 199

Vietz, Ferdinand Bernhard. *Icones Plantarum Medico-Oeconomico-Technologicarum Cum Earum Fructus Ususque Descriptione: Abbildungen Aller Medizinisch-ÖKonomisch-Technologischen GewäChse mit Der Beschreibung Ihres Gebrauches &ct..* Schalbaecher. 1804...............48, 72, 74, 92–93, 97, 108, 120–121, 124, 143, 144, 155, 158, 166–167, 180, 206–207, 210, 222

Walcott, Mary Vaux. *North American Wild Flowers.* Washington: Smithsonian Institution. 1925..........................236

Woodville, William. *Medical Botany: Containing Systematic and General Descriptions, With Plates of All the Medicinal Plants, Comprehended in the Catalogues of the Materia Medica.* London, J. Bohn. 1810–1832. .....15, 25, 33, 58, 125, 138, 160–161, 183, 188, 202, 224, 238

Yonge, Charlotte M. *The Instructive Picture Book, or, Lessons From the Vegetable World.* Edinburgh: Edmonston & Douglas. 1858. ...77

Zingiber officinale, line drawing..119

Zorn, Johannes. *Icones Plantarum Medicinalium.* Nürnberg. 1779–1790.................................44, 146–147, 214, 220

Printed in the USA
CPSIA information can be obtained
at www.ICGtesting.com
LVHW060342180424
777541LV00004B/139